DORLAND'S MEDICAL EQUIPMENT WORD BOOK FOR MEDICAL TRANSCRIPTIONISTS

D1713144

DORLAND'S MEDICAL EQUIPMENT WORD BOOK FOR MEDICAL TRANSCRIPTIONISTS

Series Editor:
SHARON B. RHODES, CMT, RHIT

Edited & Reviewed by:
Carrie Donathan, CMT

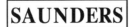

SAUNDERS
An Imprint of Elsevier Science

11830 Westline Industrial Drive
St. Louis, Missouri 63146

DORLAND'S MEDICAL EQUIPMENT WORD BOOK FOR
MEDICAL TRANSCRIPTIONISTS   0-7216-9521-3

International Standard Book Number 0-7216-9521-3

Acquisitions Editor: Karen Fabiano
Developmental Editor: Ellen Wurm
Publishing Services Manager: Peggy Fagen
Designer: Ellen Zanolle

KI/MVY
Printed in the United States of America
Last digit is the print number: 9   8   7   6   5   4   3   2   1

PREFACE

I am proud to present the *Dorland's Medical Equipment Word Book for Medical Transcriptionists*—one of the ongoing series of word books being compiled for the professional medical transcriptionist. For one hundred years, W.B. Saunders has published the *Dorland's Illustrated Medical Dictionary*. With the advent of medical transcription, it became the dictionary of choice for medical transcriptionists.

When I was approached several years ago to help develop a series of Dorland's word books for medical transcriptionists, I have to admit the thought absolutely overwhelmed me. The *Dorland's Illustrated Medical Dictionary* was one of my first book purchases when I began my transcription career over thirty years ago. To participate in this project is an honor I could never have imagined for myself!

Transcriptionists need and will continue to need trusted up-to-date resources to help them research difficult terms quickly. In developing the *Dorland's Medical Equipment Word Book for Medical Transcriptionists*, I had access to the entire Dorland's terminology database for the book's foundation. In addition to this immense database, a context editor, Carrie Donathan, CMT, a recognized leader in the field of medical transcription, was selected to review the material from the database and to remove outdated and obsolete terms. As well, Carrie spent countless hours researching terms for inclusion in this wordbook. With Carrie's extensive research and diligent work, I believe this to be the most up-to-date word book for medical equipment terms available.

In developing the medical equipment word book, I wanted the size to be manageable so the book would be easy to handle, provide a durable long-lasting binding, and use a type font large enough to read while providing extensive terminology not found in other resources available to medical transcriptionists.

Because I often would like to see what an instrument actually looks like, a separate insert of medical equipment photographs has been included in this book.

Although I have tried to produce the most thorough word book for medical equipment available to medical transcriptionists, it is difficult to include every term. New instruments and equipment are developed every day. As you discover new terms, please feel free to share them with me for inclusion in the next edition of the *Dorland's Medical Equipment Word Book for Medical Transcriptionists*.

I may be reached at the following e-mail address: Sharon@TheRhodes.com.

SHARON B. RHODES, CMT, RHIT
Brentwood, Tennessee

Aaron
    A. Cut-N-Clear disposable pencil
    A. disposable forceps
    A. epilation needle
    A. LLETZ electrode
    A. solid laparoscopic electrode

AbioCor replacement heart

Abradabloc dermabrasion instrument

abrader
    Dingman otoplasty cartilage a.
    Haverhill dermal a.
    Howard corneal a.

Abscession catheter

Absolute absorbable screw

Accolade hip prosthesis

Accufix
    A. pacemaker
    A. pacemaker lead

AccuGel
    A. impression material
    A. lens

Accugraft

AccuLength arthroplasty measuring system

Accunet embolic protection system

AccuPort seal

AccuProbe 600 cryotherapy probe

AccuRx constant flow implantable pump

Accura hydrocephalus shunt

Accurate
    A. catheter

Accurate (*continued*)
    A. Surgical and Scientific Instruments (ASSI)

Accuratome precurved papillotome

Accurus vitrectomy system

AccuStick II introducer system

AccuTrack eye-tracking system

Accuvac smoke evacuation attachment

ACE
    A. Autografter bone filter
    A. balloon
    BICAP silver A.
    A. bone screw tack
    A. Exact Torque disposable ratchet
    A. fixed-wire balloon catheter
    A. OsteoGenic Distractor (OGD) System
    A. Self-Drilling Bone Screw System
    A. spline driver
    A. surgical tray
    A. trephine bur

Ace
    A. adherent bandage
    A. aerosol cloud enhancer
    A. brace
    A. halo-cast assembly
    A. halo pelvic girdle
    A. intramedullary femoral nail system
    A. longitudinal strips dressing
    A. low-profile MR halo
    A. Mark III halo
    A. pin
    A. spica bandage
    A. Trippi-Wells tong cervical traction

Ace (*continued*)
A. Universal tong cervical
traction
A. wire tension assembly
A. wrap

Ace-Colles half ring

Ace-Fischer
A.-F. external fixator
A.-F. frame

Ace-Hershey halo jig

Ace-Hesive dressing

Ace/Normed osteodistractors

ACFS
anterior cervical plate
fixation system
Dogbone ACFS

achalasia dilator

Achieve off-pump system

Achiever
A. balloon dilatation
catheter
A. balloon dilator

Acier stainless steel suture

Ackerman
A. clip
A. lingual bar
A. needle

Ackrad
A. balloon-bearing catheter
A. Bronchitrac "L" suction
catheter
A. Cervicet dilator
A. esophageal balloon
catheter
A. H/S Elliptosphere
catheter
A. Tampa catheter set

ACL
ACL drill
ACL drill guide
ACL graft knife

Acland
A. clasp
A. clip
A. microvascular clamp
A. needle

Acland-Banis arteriotomy set

Acland-Bunke counterpressor

Acme articulator

ACMI
ACMI ACN-2 flexible
cystonephroscope
ACMI Alcock catheter
ACMI antroscope
ACMI bag
ACMI biopsy loop electrode
ACMI Bunts catheter
ACMI cautery
ACMI coated Foley catheter
ACMI cystoscopic tip
ACMI cystourethroscope
ACMI duodenoscope
ACMI Emmett hemostatic
catheter
ACMI endoscope
ACMI fiberoptic
colonoscope
ACMI fiberoptic
esophagoscope
ACMI fiberoptic
proctosigmoidoscope
ACMI flexible
sigmoidoscope
ACMI gastroscope
ACMI Marici bronchoscope
ACMI Martin endoscopic
forceps
ACMI Micro-H hysteroscope
ACMI microlens Foroblique
telescope
ACMI monopolar electrode
ACMI operating
colonoscope
ACMI Owens catheter
ACMI Pezzer drain
ACMI positive pressure
catheter

ACMI (*continued*)
   ACMI proctoscope
   ACMI resectoscope
   ACMI retrograde electrode
   ACMI severance catheter
   ACMI Thackston catheter
   ACMI Transvaginal Hydro
      laparoscope
   ACMI ulcer-measuring
      device
   ACMI ureteral catheter
   ACMI Word Bartholin gland
      catheter

Acolysis coronary probe

Acorn CorCap cardiac support
   device

acorn
   a. cannula
   a. reamer

acorn-tipped
   a.-t. bougie
   a.-t. catheter

Acquacel Hydrofiber dressing.

Acra-clip system

Acra-Cut Spiral craniotome
   blade

Acro-Flex artificial disk

AcroMed Isola Device

Acrotorque
   A. bur
   A. hand engine

AcryDerm
   A. hydrogel sheet
   A. strands
   A. strands absorbent would
      dressing

Acry Island border dressing

acrylic
   a. ball eye implant
   a. bar prosthesis
   a. cap splint

acrylic (*continued*)
   a. cement
   a. conformer eye implant
   Durabase soft rebase a.
   Durahue a.
   Duralay a.
   Dura-Liner a.
   fast-setting a.
   Flexacryl hard rebase a.
   a. graft
   a. implant material
   a. lens
   a. mold
   a. resin dressing
   Splintline a.
   TAB a.
   TJ a.
   Vita-Gel a.
   a. wafer TMJ splint

Acryl-X orthopaedic cement
   removal system

AcrySof foldable intraocular lens

ACS
   Advanced Cardiovascular
      System
   Alcon Closure System
   automated corneal shaper

ACS
   ACS Amplatz guidewire
   ACS Anchor Exchange
      device
   ACS Angioject
   ACS angioplasty catheter
   ACS angioplasty Y
      connector
   ACS balloon catheter
   ACS Concorde coronary
      dilatation catheter
   ACS Concorde OTW
      catheter
   ACS Eclipse
   ACS Endura coronary
      dilation catheter
   ACS exchange guiding
      catheter
   ACS Flowtrack-40 catheter

ACS (*continued*)
    ACS Gyroscan
    ACS Hi-Torque Balance guidewire
    ACS Hi-Torque Balance Middleweight catheter
    ACS Hi-Torque Floppy II exchange wire
    ACS Hi-Torque Iron Man guide wire
    ACS Indeflator 20/30 inflation device
    ACS JL4 French catheter
    ACS LIMA guidewire
    ACS microglide wire
    ACS Monorail perfusion balloon catheter
    ACS Multi-Link Duet coronary stent
    ACS Multi-Link OTW Duet stent
    ACS Multi-Link RX Duet stent
    ACS Multi-Link Tristar coronary stent
    ACS needle
    ACS OTW Lifestream coronary dilatation catheter
    ACS OTW Photon coronary dilatation catheter
    ACS OTW Solaris coronary dilatation catheter
    ACS percutaneous introducer
    ACS percutaneous introducer set
    ACS RX Comet coronary dilatation catheter
    ACS RX Comet VP catheter
    ACS RX Ellipse angioplasty catheter
    ACS RX Gemini catheter
    ACS RX Lifestream catheter
    ACS RX multilink stent
    ACS RX Rocket catheter
    ACS RX Solaris coronary dilatation catheter

ACS (*continued*)
    ACS RX Streak angioplasty catheter
    ACS SULP II balloon
    ACS Torquemaster catheter
    ACS Tourguide II guiding catheter
    ACS Tx2000 VP catheter
    ACS Viking catheter

ACST Tx2000 coronary dilatation catheter

ACT
    ACT MicroCoil delivery system

Acticoat silver-based burn dressing

Acticon neosphincter

Actifoam
    A. collagen sponge
    A. hemostat
    A. hemostat sponge

Actis
    A. venous flow controller
    A. venous flow device

activated balloon expandable intravascular stent

activator
    Andresen a.
    Andresen-Haupl a.
    Bimler a.
    cutout a.
    Karwetsky U-bow a.
    Klammt elastic open a.
    Metzelder modification a.
    palate-free a.
    Pfeiffer-Grobety a.
    Schmuth modification a.
    Schwarz bow-type a.
    Wunderer modification a.

Active
    A. Cath catheter

Active Life
- A. L. convex on-piece urostomy pouch with Durahesive skin barrier
- A. L. FLUSHAWAY one-piece flushable closed-end pouch system
- A. L. one-piece drainage pouch
- A. L. one-piece opaque stoma cap
- A. L. one-piece precut closed-end pouch

Activent antimicrobial ventilation tube

Activitrax
- A. single-chamber responsive pacemaker
- A. variable-rate pacemaker

ACT-one coronary stent

Actros pacemaker

actuator
NYU-Hosmer electric elbow and prehension a.

AcuBlade robotic laser

Acucair continuous airflow system

Acucise
- A. balloon
- A. cutting balloon device
- A. RP retrograde endopyelotomy catheter
- A. ureteral cutting cautery

AcuClip endoscopic multiple-clip applier

Acu-Derm
- A. IV/TPN dressing
- A. wound dressing

Acufex
- A. alignment guide
- A. arthroscope
- A. basket

Acufex (*continued*)
- A. bioabsorbable Suretac suture
- A. bioabsorbable suture anchor
- A. curved basket forceps
- A. drill
- A. drill guide
- A. Edge
- A. handle
- A. MosaicPlasty instruments
- A. rotary basket forceps
- A. rotary punch
- A. Straight basket forceps

Acufex-Suretac implant

AcuFix anterior cervical plate system

Acuflex
- A. impression material
- A. intraocular lens implant

AcuMatch
- A. L series cemented femoral stem
- A. M series modular femoral hip prosthesis

AcuMed
- A. bone graft system
- A. suture anchor
- A. tension band pin

AcuSeal cardiovascular patch

AcuSnare polypectomy device

Acuspot Sharplan Laser 710 A.

AcuTouch tissue forceps

Acutrak
- A. bone fixation system
- A. bone replacement system
- A. fusion system
- A. fusion screw
- A. Mini screw
- A. Plus screw

Acutrol suture

Acuvue
A. bifocal lens
A. disposable contact lens
A. Etafilcon A lens

Adair
A. adenotome
A. breast clamp
A. breast tenaculum
A. screw compressor
A. tissue forceps
A. tissue-holding forceps
A. uterine forceps
A.-Allis tissue forceps
A.-Veress needle

Adams
A. aspirator
A. clasp
A. kidney stone filter
A. retractor
A. rib contractor
A. saw
A.-DeWeese vena cava
     serrated clip

Adamson retractor

adapter (*also* adaptor)
Air-Lon a.
Alcock catheter a.
AMSCO Hall a.
Bard-Tuohy-Borst a.
Bernaco a.
BioLase laser a.
Brown-Roberts-Wells ring a.
butterfly a.
catheter a.
Christmas tree a.
chuck a.
C-mount a.
collet screwdriver s.
Cook plastic Luer-Lok a.
Cooper laser a.
Cordis-Dow shunt a.
Freestyle CAPD catheter a.
friction-fit a.
Grace plate 4-hold a.
Greenberg Maxi-Vise a.
halo-ring a.

adapter (*continued*)
House a.
Hudson a.
Jacobs chuck a.
Kaufman a.
Luer-Lok a.
Luer suction cannula a.
Mayfield skull clamp a.
Medi-Jector a.
Morch swivel a.
Neuroguide suction-
     irrigation a.
Nickell cystoscope a.
resectoscope a.
Rosenblum rotating a.
SACH foot a.
SafeTrak epidural catheter
     a.
Sanders ventilation a.
Sheehy-Urban sliding lens
     a.
Shiley pressure-relief a.
Storz catheter a.
Trinkle chuck a.
UAM Osteon bur a.
Universal T-a.
Venturi ventilation a.
Wullstein chuck a.
Xanar laser a.
Zeiss cine a.

Adapteur
A. multifunctional drill
     guide
A. power system

Adaptic
A. gauze
A. gauze dressing
A. nonadhering dressing

adaptor (*see* adapter)

Ada scissors

ADC Medicut shears

Adcon adhesive control gel

Add-a-Cath catheter

Add-a-Clamp

Addix needle

ADD side-directed probe

AddVent atrial-ventricular
pacemaker

adenoid
    a. curette
    a. cutter
    a. forceps
    a. punch

adenotome
    Abelson a.
    Adair a.
    a. blade
    Box a.
    Box-DeJager a.
    Breitman a.
    Cullom-Mueller a.
    Daniels a.
    guillotine a.
    Kelly direct-vision a.
    LaForce a.
    LaForce-Storz a.
    Mueller-LaForce a.
    Myles guillotine a.
    Shambaugh reverse a.
    Shulec a.
    Sluder a.
    St. Clair-Thompson a.

adhesive
    Adcon a. control gel
    ADTRA composite external
      fixator ring a.
    Aron Alpha a.
    BA bone cement a.
    bioactive bone cement a.
    Biobond tissue a.
    BioGlue
    Bond-Eze bond a.
    Brown sterile a.
    Cel Touch a.
    Coe-Pak paste a.
    Cover-Roll gauze a.
    cyanoacrylate tissue a.
    Dermabond topical skin a.
    hydroxyapatite a.

adhesive (*continued*)
    Implast bone cement a.
    Indermil tissue a.
    LiquiBand topical wound-
      closure a.
    Liquiderm liquid a.
    LPPS hydroxyapatite a.
    Mammopatch gel self a.
    methyl methacrylate
      cement a.
    Nexacryl tissue a.
    Nu-Hope a.
    Orthoset radiopaque bone
      cement a.
    Palacos cement a.
    Scanpor acrylate a.
    Silastic medical a.
    stoma cap microporous a.
    Superglue a.
    Surfit a.
    Tisseel biologic fibrogen a.
    T-Stick a.
    Urihesive expandable a.
    Zimmer low-viscosity a.

Adler
    A. attic ear punch
    A. bone forceps
    A. punch forceps
    A.-Kreutz forceps

adnexal forceps

Adson
    A. aneurysm needle
    A. angular hook
    A. arterial forceps
    A. bayonet dressing forceps
    A. bipolar forceps
    A. bone rongeur
    A. brain clip
    A. brain-exploring cannula
    A. bur
    A. cerebellar retractor
    A. clamp
    A. clip-applying forceps
    A. dural hook
    A. dural needle holder
    A. forceps with teeth

Adson (*continued*)
  A. ganglion scissors
  A. Gigli saw
  A. hemostatic forceps
  A. hypophyseal forceps
  A. laminectomy chisel
  A. microforceps
  A. monopolar forceps
  A. periosteal elevator
  A. scalp clip
  A. speculum
  A. spiral drill
  A. twist drill
  A.-Beckman retractor
  A.-Biemer forceps
  A.-Brown clamp
  A.-Brown forceps
  A.-Callison tissue forceps
  A.-Love periosteal elevator
  A.-Mixter neurosurgical
    forceps
  A.-Murphy trocar point
    needle
  A.-Rogers cranial bur
  A.-Rogers perforating drill
  A.-Vital tissue forceps

Advancit guidewire system

Advantim revision knee system

Aebli
  A. corneal scissors
  A. tenotomy scissors
  A.-Manson scissors

Aequalis humeral head implant

Aeroplast dressing

AES antiembolic stockings

Aescula lead

Aesculap
  A. alpha vessel clip
  A. argon ophthalmic laser
  A. drill
  A. excimer laser
  A. forceps
  A. needle holder
  A. skull perforator

Aesculap (*continued*)
  A. traction bow
  A. UNITRAC retraction and
    retention system
  A. Vario wound hook
    system
  A. Vascu Cut punch system

aftercataract bur

agate burnisher

AGC
  anatomic graduated
    components
      AGC Biomet total knee
        system
      AGC dual-pivot
        resection guide
      AGC Modular Tibial II
        component
      AGC porous anatomic
        femoral component
      AGC unicondylar knee
        component

Agee
  A. carpal tunnel release
    system
  A. endoscope
  A. 4-pin fixation device
  A. WristJack fracture
    reduction system

Aggressor
  A. meniscal blade
  A. meniscal shaver

Agnew
  A. canaliculus knife
  A. keratome
  A. splint
  A. tattooing needle

agraffe clamp

Agrikola
  A. eye speculum
  A. lacrimal sac retractor
  A. refractor

Agris

Agris (*continued*)
   A. rasp
   A.-Dingman submammary
      dissector

Ahlquist-Durham embolism
   clamp

AICD
   automatic implantable
      cardioverter defibrillator
   AICD-B pacemaker
   AICD-BR pacemaker
   Cadence AICD
   CPI Ventak AICD
   Guardian AICD
   AICD pacemaker
   AICD plus Tachylog device
   Res-Q AICD
   Ventak Mini II AICD
   Ventak P3 AICD

AID-B pacemaker

AIM
   AIM femoral nail system
   AIM 7 thermocouple input
      module

aimer
   Arthrotek femoral a.
   Paddu tibial a.

Ainsworth
   A. arch
   A. punch

Air-Back spinal system

air-boot
   Jobst postoperative a.-b.

Aircast
   A. Air-Stirrup leg brace
   A. Cryo Cuff
   A. fracture brace
   A. knee system
   A. pneumatic brace
   A. Swivel-Strap brace
   A. walking brace

Aire-Cuf
   A. endotracheal tube
   A. trachcostomy tube

AirFlex carpal tunnel splint

AirGEL ankle brace

Airlife
   A. cannula
   A. Dual Spray MiniSpacer
   A. MediSpacer

Airlift balloon retractor

Air-Lon
   A. adapter
   A. decannulation plug
   A. inhalation catheter
   A. laryngectomy tube
   A. tracheal tube
   A. tracheal tube brush

air-powered drill

Air-Shield-Vickers syringe tip

Airstrip composite dressing

airway
   Beck mouth tube a.
   Berman intubating
      pharyngeal a.
   binasal pharyngeal a.
   Coburg-Connell a.
   Combitube a.
   Concord/Portex a.
   Connell a.
   Foerger a.
   Guedel a.
   LMA-Unique disposable
      laryngeal mask a.
   Lumbard a.
   Luomanen oral a.
   Portex nasopharyngeal a.
   Robertazzi nasopharyngeal
      a.
   Sarfar-S a.

Akahoshi
   A. Nucleus Sustainer
   A. phaco prechopper

A-K diamond knife

Aker lens pusher

Akins valve re-do forceps

Aktusu III total artificial heart

AL-1 catheter

Alabama
>A. needle holder
>A. University forceps

Alabama-Green eye needle holder

alar
>a. cinch
>a. protector
>a. retractor
>a. screw

alar-columellar implant

Albany eye guard

Albarran
>A. bridge
>A. laser
>A. laser cystoscope
>A. lens
>A. urethroscope
>A.-Reverdin needle

Albee
>A. bone graft calipers
>A. bone saw
>A. drill
>A. olive-shaped bur
>A. orthopaedic fracture table
>A. osteotome

Albert slotted bronchoscope

Albert-Andrews laryngoscope

Albert-Smith pessary

Albizzia nail

albumin-coated vascular graft

albuminized woven Dacron tube graft

Alcatel pacemaker

Alcock
>A. bladder syringe
>A. catheter adapter

Alcock (*continued*)
>A. catheter plug
>A. hemostatic bag
>A. lithotrite
>A. obturator
>A. return-flow hemostatic catheter

Alcock-Timberlake obturator

Alcon
>A. A-OK crescent knife
>A. A-OK phacoemulsification slit knife
>A. A-OK ShortCut knife
>A. aspirator
>A. Closure System
>A. cryoextractor
>A. cryophake
>A. cryosurgical unit
>A. cystitome
>A. disposable drape
>A. I-knife
>A. indirect ophthalmoscope
>A. intraocular lens
>A. irrigating needle
>A. microsponge
>A. Phaco-Emulsifier phacoemulsification unit
>A. spatula needle
>A. suture
>A. taper-cut needle
>A. tonometer
>A. vitrectomy probe

Alden retractor

Alderkreutz tissue forceps

Aldrete needle

Aldridge rectus fascia sling

Aleman meniscotomy knife

ALERT
>A. catheter
>A. Companion II defibrillator

Alexander

Alexander (*continued*)
    A. antrostomy punch
    A. approximator
    A. bone chisel
    A. bone lever
    A. costal periosteotome
    A. dressing forceps
    A. elevator
    A. mastoid bone gouge
    A. otoplasty knife
    A perforating osteotome
    A. retractor
    A. rib raspatory
    A. tonsillar needle
    A.-Ballen orbital retractor
    A.-Farabeuf costal
      periosteotome
    A.-Farabeuf elevator
    A.-Farabeuf forceps
    A.-Matson retractor
    A.-Reiner ear syringe

Alfonso
    a. eyelid speculum
    A. guarded bur

Alfreck retractor

Alfred
    A. snare

Alger brush

AlgiDERM wound dressing

alginate wound dressing

AlgiSite alginate wound dressing

Algisorb wound dressing

Algosteril alginate dressing

aligner
    Charnley femoral inlay a.
    femoral a.
    Geo-Matt 30-degree body a.
    patellar a.
    tibial a.

alignment catheter

AL II guiding catheter

AliMed surgical drape

Alldress multilayer wound
  dressing

Allen
    A. anastomosis clamp
    A. applicator
    A. arm surgery table
    A. cecostomy trocar
    A. ePTFE ocular implant
    A. finger trap
    A. intestinal clamp
    A. intestinal forceps
    A. laparoscopic stirrups
    A. orbital implant
    A. retractor
    A. Supramid implant
    A. uterine forceps
    A. well leg holder
    A. wire threader
    A.-Barkan forceps
    A.-Barkan knife
    A.-Braley forceps
    A.-Braley intraocular lens
    A.-Braley lens implant
    A.-Brown prosthesis
    A.-Burian trabeculotome
    A.-Hanbury knife
    A.-headed screwdriver
    A.-Heffernan nasal
      speculum
    A.-Kocher clamp
    A.-Schiotz plunger retractor
      tonometer
    A.-Thorpe goniolens
    A.-Thorpe gonioscopic
      prism

Allen-type hex key

Allerdyce
    A. dissector
    A. elevator

Allergan-Humphrey
    A.-H. lensometer
    A.-H. photokeratoscope

Allergan-Simcoe C-loop
  intraocular lens

Allevyn
  A. adhesive hydrocellular
    dressing
  A. cavity dressing
  A. foam dressing
  A. hydrophilic polyurethane
    dressing
  A. Island dressing
  A. tracheostomy
    dressing

Allgower
  a. stitch
  a. suture technique

alligator
  a. clip
  a. crimper forceps
  a. cup forceps
  a. ear forceps
  a. MacCarty scissors
  a. nasal forceps

Allingham rectal speculum

Allis
  A. catheter
  A. clamp
  A. delicate tissue forceps
  A. dry dissector
  A. hemostat
  A. intestinal forceps
  A. lung retractor
  A. Micro-Line pediatric
    forceps
  A. periosteal elevator
  A. thoracic forceps
  A. tissue clamp

Allis-Abramson breast biopsy
  forceps

Allis-Adair
  A.-A. intestinal forceps
  A.-A. tissues forceps

Allis-Coakley
  A.-C. tonsillar forceps
  A.-C. tonsil-seizing
    forceps

Allis-Duval forceps

Allis-Ochsner
  A.-O. tissue forceps
  A.-O. tonsillar forceps

Allis-Willauer tissue forceps

Allison
  A. clamp
  A. lung retractor
  A. lung spatula

AlloAnchor RC

AlloDerm
  A. dermal graft
  A. processed tissue graft

allogeneic
  a. lyophilized bone graft
    implant material

allograft
  acetabular a.
  AlloGro freeze-dried bone
    a.
  a. bone vise
  bovine a.
  decalcified freeze-dried
    bone a.
  fresh frozen a.
  a.-host junction
  intercalary a.
  MTE a.
  napkin ring calcar a.
  osteoarticular a.
  Tutoplast processed a.

AlloGrip bone vise

AlloMatrix injectable putty

alloy
  Densilay a.
  Fulcast a.
  Ultracast a.
  Vera bond a.

Allport
  A. cutting bur
  A. gauze packer
  A. hook
  A. mastoid bayonet
    retractor

Allport (*continued*)
A. mastoid searcher
A. mastoid sound
A.-Babcock mastoid
searcher
A.-Babcock retractor
A.-Gifford retractor

Alm
A. clip applier
A. dilator
A. microsurgery retractor
A. self-retaining retractor

Almeida forceps

Alpar intraocular lens implant

Alpern cortex
aspirator/hydrodissector

alpha cradle

Alpha 1 penile implant

Alphatec
A. mini lag-screw system
A. small fragment system

ALR cystoresectoscope

Alta
A. cancellous screw
A. CFX reconstruction rod
A. channel bone plate
A. condylar buttress plate
A. cortical screw
A. cross-locking screw
A. distal fracture plate
A. femoral bolt
A. femoral intramedullary
rod
A. femoral plate
A. humeral rod
A. intramedullary rod
A. leg screw
A. reconstruction rod
A. supracondylar bone plate
A. supracondylar screw
A. tibial-humeral rod
A. tibial rod
A. transverse screw

Alter lip retractor

Altmann needle

Alumafoam nasal splint

Alumina cemented total hip
prosthesis

aluminum
a. cortex retractor
a. eye shield
a. fence splint
a. finger cot splint

aluminum-bronze wire suture

ALVAD artificial heart

Alvarado surgical knee holder

Alvarez-Rodriguez cardiac
catheter

Alvis
A. fixation forceps
A. foreign body eye curette
A. foreign body spud

Alvis-Lancaster sclerotome

Alway groover

Alyea vas clamp

Alzate catheter

Amazr catheter

AMBI
AMBI compression hip
screw
AMBI reamer

Ambicor
A. inflatable prosthesis
A. penile prosthesis

Ambler dilator

Ambrose
A. eye forceps
A. suture forceps

Ambu
A. bag
A. CardioPump

Ambu (*continued*)
    A. respirator

Ambu-E valve

Amcath catheter

AMC needle

AMD artificial urinary sphincter

Amdur lid forceps

Amenabar
    A. capsular forceps
    A. counterpressor
    A. iris retractor
    A. lens
    A. lens loop

Amercal intraocular lens

Amercal-Shepard intraocular
  lens

American
    A. artificial larynx
    A. Catheter Corporation
      biopsy forceps
    A. circle nephrostomy tube
    A. Endoscopy dilator
    A. Hanks uterine dilator
    A. Heyer-Schulte brain
      retractor
    A. Heyer-Schulte chin
      prosthesis
    A. Heyer-Schulte malar
      prosthesis
    A. Heyer-Schulte mammary
      prosthesis
    A. Heyer-Schulte-Radovan
      tissue expander prosthesis
    A. Heyer-Schulte
      rhinoplasty prosthesis
    A. Heyer-Schulte-Robertson
      suprapubic trocar
    A. Heyer-Schulte stent
    A. Heyer-Schulte testicular
      prosthesis
    A. Heyer-Schulte T-tube
    A. Medical Optics Baron
      lens

American (*continued*)
    A. Medical Source
      laparoscope
    A. Optical Cardiocare
      pacemaker
    A. Optical coagulator
    A. Optical ophthalmometer
    A. Optical photocoagulator
    A. silk suture
    A. umbilical scissors
    A. vascular stapler
    A. wire gauge

Amersham
    A. CDCS A-type needle
    A. J. tube

Amerson bone elevator

Ames ventriculoperitoneal shunt

Amico
    A. chisel
    A. drill

Amko vaginal speculum

AMK total knee system

AML total hip prosthesis

Amnihook amniotic membrane
  perforator

amnioscope
    Erosa a.
    Saling a.

amniotome
    Baylor a.
    Beacham a.
    Glove-n-Gel a.

AMO
    Allergan Medical Optics
      AMO Advent contact
        lens
      AMO Array foldable
        intraocular lens
      AMO lensometer
      AMO
        phacoemulsification
        lens-folder forceps

AMO (*continued*)
   Allergan (*continued*)
      AMO photokeratoscope
      AMO Prestige
        advanced cataract
        extraction system
      AMO scleral implant
      AMO Sensar intraocular
        lens
      AMO Series 4 phaco
        handpiece
      AMO vitreous
        aspiration cutter

Amoils
  A. cryoextractor
  A. cryopencil
  A. cryophake
  A. cryoprobe
  A. cryosurgical unit
  A. iris retractor
  A. probe
  A. refractor

AMO-PhacoFlex lens and
  inserter

AMO-Prestige phaco system

AmpErase electrocautery

Amplatz
  A. anchor system
  A. angiography needle
  A. aortography catheter
  A. cardiac catheter
  A. Clot Buster
  A. fascial dilator
  A. femoral catheter
  A. goose neck snare
  A. Hi-Flo torque-control
    catheter
  A. injector
  A. left I, II catheter
  A. microsnare
  A. retinal snare
  A. sheath
  A. Super Stiff guidewire
  A. thrombectomy device
    (Clot Buster)

Amplatz (*continued*)
  A. torque wire
  A. TractMaster system
  A. tube guide
  A. ventricular septal defect
    device

Amplex guidewire

amputation
  a. knife
  a. retractor
  a. saw
  a. screw

AMS
  AMS Ambicore penile
    prosthesis
  AMS autoclavable
    laparoscope
  AMS Coaguloop
  AMS CX penile prosthesis
    cylinder
  AMS disposable trocar
  AMS Endoview camera
  AMS Hydroflex penile
    prosthesis
  AMS SPARC sling system
  AMS Sphincter 800 urinary
    prosthesis
  AMS ureteral stent

AMSCO
  AMSCO Hall adapter
  AMSCO headholder
  AMSCO hysteroscope
  AMSCO Orthairtome drill

Amset
  A. ALPS
  A. ALPS anterior locking
    plate system
  A. R-F fixation system
  A. R-F rod
  A. R-F screw

Amsler
  A. aqueous transplant
    needle
  A. scleral marker

Amsterdam biliary stent

Amstutz
  A. cemented hip prosthesis
  A. femoral component
  A. total hip replacement

Amstutz-Wilson osteotomy

Amtech-Killeen pacemaker

Amussat probe

anal
  a. dilator
  a. retractor
  a. speculum

Anastaflo
  A. intravascular shunt
  A. stent

Anastasia bougie

Anastomark flexible coronary
  graft marker

anastomosis
  a. apparatus
  a. clamp
  a. forceps
  Martin-Gruger a.

anatomic
  a. graduated components
  a. hip system
  a. medullary locking total
    system
  porous-coated a.
  a. Precoat hip prosthesis

Anatomic/Intracone reamer

Ancap braided silk suture

anchor
  Acufex bioabsorbable
    suture a.
  Acumed suture a.
  Arthrex FASTak suture a.
  a. band
  a. plate
  AxyaWeld bone a.
  Bio-Anchor suture a.

anchor (continued)
  Bio-Fastak suture/a.
  Biologically Quiet suture a.
  Bio-Phase suture a.
  BioROC EZ suture a.
  BioSphere suture a.
  Bone Bullet suture a.
  Catera suture a.
  Corkscrew suture a.
  DRG Sherlock threaded
    suture a.
  a. endosteal implant
  E-Z ROC a.
  FASTak suture a.
  FastIn threaded a.
  Hall sacral a.
  Harpoon suture a.
  a. hook
  Innovasive Devices ROC SX
    suture a.
  Isola spinal implant system
    a.
  Kurer a,.
  Lemoine-Searcy a.
  Mainstay urologic soft tissue
    a.
  mini Bio-Phase suture a.
  Mitek absorbable bone a.
  Mitek Fastin threaded a.
  Mitek GII Easy A.
  Mitek GII suture a,.
  Mitek GL a.
  Mitek Knotless a.
  Mitek Ligament a.
  Mitek Micro a.
  Mitek Minim GII a.
  Mitek Mini GLS a.
  Mitek Panalot a.
  Mitek rotator cuff a.
  Mitek Tacit threaded a.
  a. needle holder
  Ogden soft tissue to bone a.
  PaBA a.
  Panalok absorbable a.
  Panalok RC QuickAnchor
    Plus suture a.
  Parachute Corkscrew
    suture a.

anchor (*continued*)
    PeBA a.
    Radix a.
    Revo suture a.
    ROC XS suture a.
    a. screw
    Searcy fixation a.
    Sherlock threaded suture a.
    SmartAnchor-D suture a.
    SmartAnchor-L suture a.
    a. soft tissue biopsy device
    a. splint
    Statak suture a.
    Stryker wedge suture a.
    a. surgical needle
    Tacit threaded a.
    TAG Rod II suture a.
    traction a.
    UltraFix a.
    UltraSorb suture a
    Zest Anchor Advanced
      Generation (ZAAG) bone
      anchor

anchored catheter

anchor/fixation
    Search a./f.

anchoring peg

Anchorlok soft tissue anchor

anchor/Snap-Pak
    Mitek Panalot RC a./S.-P.

Ancrofil clasp wire

Ancure
    A. bifurcated system
    A. balloon catheter system
    A. stent-graft
    A. tube system

Andersen mercury-weighted
  tube

Anderson
    A. acetabular prosthesis
    A. biopsy punch
    A. clamp
    A. columellar prosthesis

Anderson (*continued*)
    A. converse iris scissors
    A. curette
    A. distractor
    A. double ball
    A. double-end knife
    A. double-end retractor
    A. elevator
    A. flexible suction tube
    A. nasal strut
    A. splint
    A. suture pusher and
      double hook
    A. traction bow
    A.-Adson self-retaining
      retractor
    A.-Neivert osteotome

Ando
    A. aortic clamp
    A. motor-driven probe

Andre hook

Andrews
    A. applicator
    A. chisel
    A. comedo extractor
    A. gouge
    A. mastoid gouge
    A. osteotome
    a. spinal frame
    A. suction tip
    A. tonsillar forceps
    A. tonsil-seizing forceps
    A. tracheal retractor
    A.-Hartmann forceps
    A.-Hartmann rongeur
    A.-Pynchon suction tube

AnEber probe

Anel
    A. lacrimal probe
    A. syringe

aneurysm
    a. clamp
    a. clip
    a. clip applier
    a. forceps

aneurysm (*continued*)
    a. neck dissector
    a. needle

AneuRx
    A. aortic aneurysm stent-
      graft
    A. DTA stent graft system
    A. IDS delivery system

AngeCool RF catheter ablation
  system

AngeFix lead

AngeFlex lead

AngeLase combined mapping-
  laser probe

Angell
    A. curette
    A. gauze packer
    A.-James dissector
    A.-James hypophysectomy
      forceps
    A.-James punch forceps
    A.-Shiley bioprosthetic heart
      valve
    A.-Shiley xenograft
      prosthetic valve

AngePass lead system

Angestat hemostasis introducer

Angetear tear-away introducer

Angiocath
    A. flexible catheter
    a. PRN catheter

angiocatheter
    Brockenbrough a.
    Corlon a.
    Deseret a.
    Eppendorf a.
    Mikro-Tip a.
    a. with looped
      polypropylene suture

Angiocor
    a. prosthetic valve
    a. rotational thrombolizer

Angioflow high-flow catheter

angiographic
    a. balloon occlusion
      catheter
    a. portacaval shunt

angiography
    a. catheter
    a. needle

Angioguard catheter device

AngioJet
    A. catheter
    A. rapid thrombectomy
      system
    A. rheolytic thrombectomy
      system
    A. saline jet-vacuum device
      catheter
    A. thrombectomy catheter

Angio-Kit catheter

angiolaser
    pulsed a.

Angiomedics catheter

AngioOPTIC microcatheter

angiopigtail catheter

angioplasty
    a. balloon
    a. balloon catheter
    a. guiding catheter
    a. sheath

angioscope
    Baxter a.
    Coronary Imagecath a.
    flexible a.
    Imagecath rapid exchange
      a.
    Masy a.
    Mitsubishi a.
    Olympus a.
    Optiscope a.

angioscopic valvulotome

Angio-Seal

Angio-Seal (*continued*)
   A. catheter
   A. hemostasis system
   A. hemostatic puncture
     closure device

AngioStent stent

angiotribe
   Ferguson a.
   a. forceps
   Zweifel a.

AngioVista angiographic system

angle
   a. port pump
   a. splint

angled
   a. ball-end electrode
   a. balloon catheter
   a. biter
   a. capsular forceps
   a. clip
   a. counterpressor
   a. DeBakey clamp
   a. decompression retractor
   a. discission hook
   a. guidewire
   a. iris retractor
   a. iris spatula
   a. lens loop
   a. nucleus removal loop
   a. peripheral vascular
     clamp
   a. pigtail catheter
   a. pleural tube
   a. probe
   a. ring curette
   a. scissors
   a. stone forceps
   a. vein retractor

Angle-Pezzer drain

angle-tip
   a.-t. electrode
   a.-t. Glidewire
   a.-t. guidewire
   a.-t. urethral catheter

Angstrom MD implantable
   single-lead cardioverter-
   defibrillator

angular
   a. elevator
   a. knife
   a. needle
   a. scissors

angulated
   a. catheter
   a. iris spatula

Anis
   A. aspirating cannula
   A. ball reverse-curvature
     capsular polisher
   A. capsulotomy forceps
   A. corneal forceps
   A. corneal scissors
   A. corneoscleral forceps
   A. disk capsular polisher
   A. intraocular lens forceps
   A. irrigating vectis
   A. microforceps
   A. microsurgical tying
     forceps
   A. needle holder
   A. staple lens
   A. straight corneal forceps
   A. tying forceps
   A.-Barraquer needle holder

Ankeney sternal retractor

ankle
   a. air stirrup
   a. rehab pump
   a. weight

Ann Arbor
   A. A. phrenic retractor
   A. A. towel clamp

ANNE anesthesia infuser

annular
   a. detector
   a. gouge

AnnuloFlex annuloplasty ring

anoscope
Bacon a.
Bensaude a.
Bodenheimer a.
Boehm a.
Brinkerhoff a.
Buie-Hirschman a.
Burnett a.
Disposo-Scope a.
Fansler a.
Fansler-Ives a.
fiberoptic a.
Goldbacher a.
Hirschman a.
Ives al.
Ives-Fansler a.
KleenSpec disposable a.
Muer a.
Munich-Crosstreet a.
Otis a.
Pratt a.
Proscope a.
Pruitt a.
rotating speculum a.
Sims a.
Sklar a.
slotted a.
Smith a.
speculum a.
Welch Allyn a.

anosigmoidoscope

Anspach
A. cranial perforator
A. craniotome
A. diamond dissecting
cutter
A. 65K drill
A. 65K instrument
system
A. leg holder

antegrade
a. internal stent
a. ureteral stent
a. valvulotome

antegrade/retrograde
compression nail

anterior
a. capsule forceps
a. cervical plate fixation
system
a. chamber acrylic implant
a. chamber intraocular lens
a. chamber irrigating
cannula
a. chamber irrigating vectis
a. chamber irrigator
a. chamber maintainer
a. chamber synechia
scissors
a. chamber tube shunt
encircling band
a. commissure
laryngoscope
a. commissure
microlaryngoscope
a. cruciate ligament drill
guide
a. crurotomy nipper
a. footplate pick
a. prostatic rectractor
a. resection clamp
a. segment forceps

anterior-posterior
a.-p. cutting block
a.-p. cystoresectoscope

Anthony
A. aspirating tube
A. cast boot
A. elevator
A. enucleation compressor
A. gorget
A. mastoid suction tube
A. orbital compressor
A. pillar retractor
A. quadrisected dilator
A. suction tube
A.-Fisher antral balloon
A.-Fisher forceps

Anthron
A. II catheter
A. heparinized catheter

anthropometric total hip

antibiotic-coated stent

anticavitation drill

antimicrobial
a. catheter
a. removal device

antirotation guide

antisiphon valve

antitachycardia pacemaker

Antoni-Hook lumbar puncture
cannula

antral
a. balloon
a. bur
a. chisel
a. curette
a. drain
a. forceps
a. gouge
a. irrigator
a. perforator
a. punch
a. rasp
a. retractor
a. sinus cannula
a. trocar
a. trocar needle

Antron catheter

antroscope
ACMI a.
Nagashima right-angle a.
Reichert a.

antrum-exploring needle

anvil
Bunnell a.

Anzio catheter

AO
ankle orthosis

AO
AO blade plate
AO cancellous screw
AO condylar blade plate

AO (*continued*)
AO contoured T plate
AO cortex screw
AO drill bit
AO dynamic compression
plate
AO femoral distractor
AO gouge
AO guidepin
AO hook plate
AO internal fixator
AO lag screw
AO plate bender
AO reconstruction plate
AO reduction forceps
AO semitubular plate
AO slotted medullary nail
AO small fragment plate
AO spinal internal fixation
AO spongiosa screw
AO spoon plate
AO stopped-drill guide
AO tap
AO tension band

AO/ASIF orthopaedic implant

AOO pacemaker

AOR
A. check traction device
A. collateral ligament
retractor

aortic
a. aneurysm clamp
a. aneurysm forceps
a. arch cannula
a. balloon pump
a. bioprosthetic valve
a. cannula clamp
a. catheter
a. connector system
a. curette
a. dilator
a. director ellipse cannula
a. occluder
a. occlusion clamp
a. occlusion forceps
a. perfusion cannula

aortic (*continued*)
   a. punch
   a. root perfusion needle
   a. sump tube
   a. tube graft
   a. valve retractor

aortography
   a. catheter
   a. needle

aortopulmonary shunt

A-P cutting block

Apex pin

Apexo elevator

Apfelbaum
   A. bipolar forceps
   A. cerebellar retractor
   A. micromirror

APF Moore-type femoral stem

API osteotome

apicitis curette

apicoaortic
   a. conduit heart valve
   a. shunt heart valve

apicolysis retractor

Apligraf
   A. graft
   A. Graftskin
   A. skin graft material
   A. venous ulcer graft
      material

Apollo
   A. hip prosthesis
   A. knee prosthesis
   A. 3 triple-lumen
      papillotome

A-Port
   A. implantable port
   A. vascular access

apparatus
   biphase Morris fixation a.

apparatus (*continued*)
   Brawley suction a.
   Buck convoluted traction a.
   Buck extension a.
   C-arm fluoroscopic a.
   cryosurgical a.
   Davidson pneumothorax a.
   fixation a.
   Frac-Sur a.
   fracture-banding a.
   halo a.
   Heyns abdominal
      decompression a.
   Hilal embolization a.
   Horsley-Clarke stereotactic
      a.
   Kandel stereotactic a.
   Killian suspension gallows
      a.
   Kirschner traction a.
   Kuntscher traction a.
   Lynch suspension a.
   Mayfield-Kees skull fixation
      a.
   McKesson pneumothorax a.
   Parham-Martin fracture a.
   Ruth-Hedwig
      pneumothorax a.
   Sayre suspension a.
   Semm pneumoperitoneum
      a.
   Stryker Constavac closed-
      wound suction a.
   suction a.
   Vactro perilimbal suction a.

appendage clamp

appendectomy clamp

appendiceal retractor

applanator
   Johnston LASIK flap a.

Apple
   A. laparoscopic stone
      grabber
   A. Medical bipolar forceps
   A. trocar

appliance
- arch bar facial fracture a.
- biphasic pin a.
- Bradford fracture a.
- Buck fracture a.
- craniofacial fracture a.
- Dewald halo spinal a.
- Erich facial fracture a.
- extraoral fracture a.
- Frac-Sur a.
- Gerster fracture a.
- Goldthwait fracture a.
- Hibbs fracture a.
- intraoral fracture a.
- Janes fracture a.
- Jelenko facial fracture a.
- Jewett fracture a.
- Joseph septal fracture a.
- Mitek anchor a.
- obturator a.
- Roger Anderson pin fixation a,.
- SACH orthopaedic a.
- vasocillator fracture a.
- Whitman fracture a.
- Wilson fracture a.
- Winter facial fracture a.

applicator
- Absolok endoscopic clip a.
- Cohen suture a.
- colpostat a.
- Falope-ring a.
- Farrior suction a.
- Filshie clip minilaparotomy a.
- a. forceps
- Kevorkian-Younge uterine a.
- Mayfield clip a.
- minilaparotomy Falope-ring a.
- Montrose dressing a.
- multifire clip a.
- multiload occlusive clip a.
- resorbable thread clip a.
- ring a.

Applied Medical mini ureteroscope

applier
- AcuClip endoscopic multiple-clip a.
- Advanced Surgical suture a.
- Alm clip a.
- aneurysm clip a.
- Autoclip a.
- automatic Hemoclip a.
- Auto Suture Clip-A-Matic clip a.
- bayonet clip a.
- clip a.
- Crockard transoral clip a.
- Endo Clip a.
- Gam-Mer clip a.
- Hamby right-angle clip a.
- Heifitz clip a.
- hemostatic clip a.
- Hulka clip a.
- Kaufman clip a.
- Kees clip a.
- Kerr clip a.
- LDS clip a.
- Ligaclip MCA multiple-clip a.
- Malis clip a.
- Mayfield miniature clip a.
- Mayfield temporary aneurysm clip a.
- McFadden Vari-Angle clip a.
- mini a.
- Mount-Olivecrona clip a.
- Mt. Clemens Hospital clip a.
- Multifire Endo hernia clip a.
- multiloaded clip a.
- Olivecrona clip a.
- pivot clip a.
- Raney scalp clip a.
- Right Clip a.
- Sano clip a.
- Schwartz clip a.
- Scoville clip a.
- Scoville-Drew clip a.
- Spetzler clip a.
- Sugita jaws clip a.
- surgical clip a.
- Vari-Angle McFadden clip a.

applier (*continued*)
    vascular clip a.
    Weck clip a.
    Yasargil clip a.
    Zmurkiewicz clip. a.

Appose skin stapler

approximation forceps

approximator
    Allerdyce a.
    Christoudias a.
    Ikuta clamp a.
    Iwashi clamp a.
    Kleinert-Kutz clamp a.
    Microspike a.
    Neuromeet nerve a.
    Neuromeet soft tissue a.
    Wolvek sternal a.

A-Probe
    Soft-Touch A.

Aquacel Hydrofiber wound dressing

Aquaflex contact lens

Aquaflo hydrogel wound dressing

Aquamatic dressing

Aquaphor
    A. gauze
    A. gauze dressing

Aquaplast
    A. cast
    A. mold
    A. splint
    A. tie-down dressing

Aqua-Purator suction device

Aquasorb
    A. border with Covaderm tape
    A. transparent hydrogel dressing

aqueous
    a. transplant needle

aqueous (*continued*)
    a. tube shunt

arachnoid
    a. Beaver blade
    a. knife

arachnoid-shaped blade

arachnophlebectomy needle

Arani double-loop guiding catheter

Arbuckle-Shea trocar

Arbuckle sinus probe

Arc-22 catheter

arch
    a. bar cutter
    a. bar facial fracture appliance
    FemoStop femoral artery compression a.
    a. rake retractor

Archer splinter forceps

archimedean drill

archwire
    Jarabak-type a.

Arco
    A. atomic pacemaker
    A. lithium pacemaker

arcuate skin stapler

Arem-Madden retractor

Arem retractor

Arenberg
    A. dural palpator elevator
    A. endolymphatic sac knife

Arenberg-Denver inner-ear valve implant

Arglaes wound dressing

argon
    a. blue laser
    a.-fluoride laser

argon (*continued*)
a. gas anticoagulator
a. green laser
a. guidewire
a.-krypton laser
a. ion laser
a. laser photocoagulator
a. plasma coagulator
a. pump dye laser
a. vessel dilator

Argyle
A. anti-reflux valve
A. arterial catheter
A. chest tube
A. CPAP nasal cannula
A. endotracheal tube
A. Medicut R. catheter
A. oxygen catheter
A. Penrose tubing
A. Sentinel Seal chest tube
A. silicon Salem sump
a. trocar
A. trocar catheter
A. umbilical vessel catheter

Aria
A. CABG
A. prosthetic coronary artery bypass graft

Arkan sharpening-stone needle

Arlt
A. fenestrated lens scoop
A. lens loupe

Armstrong
A. beveled grommet drain tube
A. beveled grommet myringotomy tube
A. ventilation tube
A. V9-Vent tube

Army
A. bone gouge
A. chisel
A. osteotome

Army-Navy retractor

Arnoff external fixation device

Arnott
A. dilator
A. one-piece all-PMMA intraocular lens

Aronson
A. esophageal retractor
A. lateral sternomastoid retractor
A.-Fletcher antrum cannula

Array multifocal intraocular lens

Arrequi
A. KPL laparoscopic knot pusher
A. laparoscopic knot pusher ligator

Arrow
A. AutoCAT intraaortic balloon pump
A. articulation paper forceps
A. balloon wedge catheter
A. Berman angiographic balloon
A. Blue FlexTip
A. Flex intraaortic balloon catheter
A. FlexTip Plus catheter
A. LionHeart left ventricular assist system
A. Multi-Lumen Access Catheter (MAC)
A. PICC
A. pullback atherectomy catheter
A. pulmonary artery catheter
A. QuadPolar electrode catheter
A. QuickFlash arterial catheter
A. Raulerson introducer syringe
A. sheath

Arrow (*continued*)
  A. TheraCath epidural
    catheter
  A TransAct intraortic
    balloon pump
  A. true torque wire guide
  A. tube
  A. TwinCath multilumen
    peripheral catheter
  A. two-lumen hemodialysis
    catheter
  A.-Berman angiographic
    balloon
  A.-Berman balloon catheter
  A.-Fischell EVAN needle
  A.-Howes multilumen
    catheter
  A.-Howes quad-lumen
    catheter
  A.-Trerotola percutaneous
    thrombolytic device

ArrowFlex
  A. intraaortic balloon
    catheter
  A. sheath

ArrowGard
  A. Blue antiseptic-coated
    catheter
  A. Blue central venous
    catheter
  A. Blue Line catheter

Arrowsmith
  A. corneal marker
  A. fixation forceps

Arrowsmith-Clerf pin-closing
  forceps

Arroyo
  A. forceps
  A. trephine

Arruga
  A. curved capsular forceps
  A. extraction hook
  A. eye retractor
  A. speculum
  A. eye trephine

Arruga (*continued*)
  A. globe retractor
  A. globe speculum
  A. lacrimal trephine
  A. lens
  A. lens expressor
  A. needle holder
  A.-Gill forceps
  A.-McCool capsular forceps

ArtAssist compression dressing

Artec balloon catheter

Artegraft collagen vascular graft

arterial
  a. cannula
  a. clamp
  a. embolectomy catheter
  a. filter
  a. forceps
  a. graft prosthesis
  a. irrigation catheter
  a. needle
  a. silk suture

arteriography needle

arteriotomy scissors

arteriovenous catheter

Arthrex
  A. arthroscope
  A. Bio-Corkscrew suture
    anchor
  A. Bio-FASTak suture anchor
  A. Bio-Transfix cross pin
    fixation
  A. coring reamer
  A. drill guide
  A. FASTak suture anchor
  A. FiberWire suture
  A. OATS bone plug
  A. sheathed interference
    screw
  A. tibial tunnel guide
  A. TissueTak II
    bioabsorbable implant
  A. Transfix II cross pin
    fixation
  A. zebra pin

ArthroCare
 A. arthroscopic system
 A. Rubo-Vac device
 A. thermal wand

Arthrofile orthopaedic rasp

Arthro Force
 A. F. basket cutting forceps
 A. F. hook scissors

Arthro-Lok
 A.-L. knife
 A.-L. system of Beaver
  blades

arthroscope
 Acufex a.
 Arthrex a.
 Baxter angled a.
 Circon a.
 Citscope a.
 Codman a.
 Concept Intravision a.
 Downs a.
 Dyonics rod lens a.
 Eagle straight-ahead a.
 examining a.
 fiberoptic a.
 Flexiscope a.
 Hopkins a.
 Lumina rod lens a.
 4M 30-degree a.
 O'Connor operating a.
 Panoview a.
 Richard Wolf a.
 Sapphire View a.
 spinal a.
 Storz a.
 Stryker a.
 Takagi a.
 Watanabe a.
 Wolf a.
 Zimmer a.

arthroscopic
 a. ankle holder
 a. banana blade
 a. cannula
 a. knife

arthroscopic (*continued*)
 a. leg holder
 a. osteotome
 a. probe
 a. punch
 a. scissors
 a. shaver
 a. sheath
 a. synovector

Arthroscrew arthroscopic
 suturing device

ArthroSew suturing system

Arthrotek
 A. calibrated cylinder
 A. Ellipticut hand
  instruments
 A. femoral aimer
 A. tibial fixation device

arthrotome
 Hall a.

ArthroWand
 CAPS a.

articulated external fixator

articulating paper forceps

Arti-holder tweezers

Artilk forceps

Artisan
 A. phakic intraocular lens
 A. wide-angle vaginal
  speculum

Artmann
 A. disarticulation chisel
 A. elevator
 A. raspatory

ARUM Colles fixation pin

ASAP
 ASAP automated biopsy
  system
 ASAP channel cut
  automated biopsy
  needle

ASAP (*continued*)
  ASAP PinPoint guiding
    introducer needle
  ASAP prostate biopsy
    needle
  ASAP Stacker automated
    multi-sample biopsy
    system

Ascension
  MCP
    (metacarpophalangeal)
    total joint
  PIP (proximal
    interphalangeal) total joint

Ascent catheter

Asch
  A. clamp
  A. nasal clamp
  A. septal forceps
  A. septal straightener
  A. septal-straightening
    forceps
  A. uterine secretion scoop

Ascon instruments

Asepto
  A. bulb syringe
  A. suction tube

Ash
  A. catheter
  A. dental forceps
  A. septum-straightening
    forceps

Ashbell hook

Ashby fluoroscopic foreign body
  forceps

Asherman chest seal

Ashley
  A. breast prosthesis
  A. cleft palate elevator
  A. retractor

ASICO multi-angled diamond
  knife

ASIF
  ASIF broad dynamic
    compression bone plate
  ASIF screw pin
  ASIF T plate
  ASIF twist drill

ASI uroplasty TCU dilatation
  catheter

Aslan
  A. endoscopic scissors
  A. 2-mm minilaparoscope
  a. needle holder

Asnis
  A. guided screw
  A. 2 guided screw
  A. III cannulated screw
  A. pin

aspirating
  a. cannula
  a. curette
  a. dissector
  a. needle
  a. syringe
  a. tube

aspiration
  a. apparatus
  a. biopsy needle

aspirator
  Alcon a.
  Aspirette endocervical a.
  bronchoscopic a.
  Broyles a.
  Care-e-Vac portable a.
  Castroviejo orbital a.
  Cavitron a.
  Clerf a.
  Cogsell tip a.
  DeLee meconium trap a.
  DeVilbiss Vacu-Aide a.
  Dieulafoy a.
  Egnell uterine a.
  Endo-Assist sponge a.
  endocervical a.
  endometrial a.
  Fink cataract a.

aspirator (*continued*)
Frazier suction tip a.
gallbladder a.
Gomco uterine a.
Gottschalk middle ear a.
Gradwohl sternal bone
marrow a.
GynoSampler endometrial
a.
Hydrojette a.
Kelman a.
Leasure a.
Monoject bone marrow a.
Stedman suction pump a.
Thorek gallbladder a.
Tompkins a.
Universal a.
uterine a.
Vent-O-Vac a.

aspirator/hydrodissector
Alpern cortex a.

Aspirette endocervical aspirator

Aspir-Vac probe

ASR
ASR blade
ASR scalpel

ASSI
ASSI bipolar coagulating
forceps
ASSI breast dissector
ASSI cannula
ASSI cranial blade
ASSI Microspike
approximator clamp
ASSI wire pass drill

Assistant Free
A. F. retractor
A. F. Stulberg leg positioner
A. F. suture

Aston
A. facelift scissors
A. nasal retractor
A. submental retractor

Astra pacemaker

Astro-Trace Universal adapter
clip

Asuka PTCA catheter

Aten olecranon screw

Athens
A. forceps
A. suture spreader

atherectomy
a. catheter
a. device

AtheroCath
A. Bantam coronary
atherectomy catheter
DVI Simpson A.
A. GTO coronary
atherectomy catheter
Simpson coronary A.
Simpson peripheral A.
A. spinning blade catheter

Atkins
A. esophagoscopic
telescope
A. nasal splint
A. tonsillar knife

Atkins-Cannard tracheotomy
tube

Atkinson
A. corneal scissors
A. endoprosthesis
A 325-G short curved
cystitome
A. introducer
A. keratome
A. retrobulbar needle
A. sclerotomy
A. single-bevel blunt-tip
needle
A. tip peribulbar needle
A. tube stent

Atkinson-Walker scissors

Atlantic ileostomy catheter

Atlantis SR coronary intravascular
ultrasound catheter

atlas
- a. LP PTCA balloon dilatation catheter
- a. ULP PTCA balloon dilatation catheter

Atlee
- A. bronchus clamp
- A. uterine dilator

A-Trac atraumatic clamping system

Atrac-II double-balloon catheter

Atrac multipurpose balloon catheter

Atra-Grip clamp

Atraloc needle

Atrauclip
- A. grip clamp
- A. hemostatic clip

atraumatic
- a. braided silk suture
- a. chromic suture
- a. curved grasper
- a. intestinal clamp
- a. needle
- a. tissue forceps
- a. visceral forceps

Atraumax peripheral vascular clamp

atrial
- a. cannula
- a. clamp
- a. demand-inhibited pacemaker
- a. demand-triggered pacemaker
- a. electrode
- a. pacing wire
- a. septal defect single disk closure device
- a. septal retractor
- a. synchronous ventricular-inhibits pacemaker
- a. tracking pacemaker

atrial (*continued*)
- a. triggered ventricular-inhibited pacemaker
- a. and ventricular implantable cardioverter defibrillator

Atrial View Ventak implantable cardioverter-defibrillator

Atricor Cordis pacemaker

atrioseptostomy catheter

Atrium hemodialysis graft

attic
- a. cannula
- a. dissector
- a. hook

Aufranc
- A. arthroplasty gouge
- A. cobra retractor
- A. cup
- A. dissector
- A. femoral neck retractor
- A. finishing ball reamer
- A. finishing cup reamer
- A. hip retractor
- A. hook
- A. offset reamer
- A. periosteal elevator
- A. psoas retractor
- A. push retractor
- A. trochanteric awl

Aufricht
- A. elevator
- A. glabellar rasp
- A. nasal rasp
- A. nasal retractor
- A. scissors
- A. septal speculum
- A.-Lipsett nasal rasp

auger wire

Ault intestinal clamp

aural
- a. forceps
- a. magnifier

aural (*continued*)
    a. speculum

auricular
    a. appendage catheter
    a. appendage clamp
    a. appendage forceps
    a. prosthesis

Austin
    A. attic dissector
    A. awl
    A. clip
    A. dissection knife
    A. duckbill elevator
    A. excavator
    A. footplate elevation
    A. forceps
    A. needle
    A. oval curette
    A. piston
    A. right-angle elevator
    A. sickle knife
    A. strut calipers

Austin Moore
    A. M. bone reamer
    A. M. corkscrew
    A. M. curved
       endoprosthesis
    A. M. extractor
    A. M. inside-outside calipers
    A. M. mortising chisel
    A. M.–Murphy bone skid
    A. M. pin
    A. M. rasp
    A. M. straight-stem
       endoprosthesis

Auth
    A. atherectomy catheter
    A. knife

Auto-Band Steri-Drape drape

AutoCat intra-aortic balloon
   pump

Autoclip
    A. applier
    Totco A.

autofunduscope

autologous
    a. fibrin tissue adhesive
    a. stem

automatic
    a. catheter
    a. cranial drill
    a. Hemoclip applier
    a. needle driver
    a. ratchet snare
    a. screwdriver
    a. skin retractor
    a. stapling device
    a. suction device
    a. tourniquet

autoperfusion
    a. balloon
    a. balloon catheter

autopsy
    a. blade
    a. handle

Autostat
    A. hemostatic clip
    A. ligating clip

Auto Suture
    A. S. ABBI system
    A. S. clip
    A. S. Clip-A-Matic clip applier
    A. S. curette
    A. S. device
    A Suture endoscopic
       suction-irrigation device
    A. S. forceps
    A. S. Mini-CABG occlusion
       clamp
    A. S. Multifire Endo GIA 30
       stapler
    A. S. One-Shot anastomotic
       device
    A. S. Premium CEEA stapler
    A. S. Soft Thoracoport
    A. S. SurgiStitch
    A. S. Soft Thoracoport
    A. S. surgical mesh
    A. S. surgical stapler

Autosyringe pump

autotome drill

Auvard
A. Britetrac speculum
A. clamp
A. cranioclast
A. weighted vaginal
retractor
A. weighted vaginal
speculum
A.-Remine vaginal
speculum
A.-Zweifel forceps

AV
AV DeClot catheter
AV fistula needle
AV Gore-Tex graft
AV junctional pacemaker
AV sequential demand
pacemaker
AV synchronous pacemaker

AVA 3Xi venous access device

Avalox skin clip

Avanti introducer

AVCO aortic balloon

AVE
AVE GFX coronary stent
AVE Micro stent

Avenida
Avenida dilator
A.-Torres dilator

Avina female urethral plug

Avitene
A. hemostatic material
A. microfibrillar collage
hemostat

AV-Paceport thermodilution
catheter

awl
Aufranc trochanteric a.
Austin a.

awl (*continued*)
bone a.
Carroll a.
Carter-Rowe a.
curved a.
DePuy a.
Ferran a.
Kelsey-Frey bone a.
Kirklin sternal a.
lacrimal a.
Mustarde a.
Obwegeser a.
pointed a.
reamer a.
rectangular a.
rib brad a.
Rochester a.
Rush pin reamer a.
starter a.
Stedman a.
sternal perforating a.
Swanson scaphoid a.
T-handle bone a.
trochanteric a.
Uniflex distal targeting a.
Wangensteen a.
Wilson a.
wire-passing a.
Zelicof orthopaedic a.
Zuelzer a.

Axcis percutaneous myocardial
revascularization (PMR)
system

Axenfeld nerve loop

Axhausen needle holder

axillary catheter

Axiom
A. DG balloon angioplasty
catheter
A. drain

axis-traction forceps

Axius off-pump system

Axxcess ureteral catheter

Axxess spinal cord stimulator

Axya bone anchor system and kit (BAK)

AxyaWeld
A. bone anchor
A. instrument
A. J-tip suture welding system

Ayers
A. chalazion forceps
A. spatula

Ayerst instruments

Aylesbury cervical spatula

Ayre
A. brush
A. cervical spatula

Ayre (*continued*)
A. cone knife
A. tube

Ayre-Scott cervical cone knife

Azar
A. corneal scissors
A. cystitome
A. intraocular forceps
A. iris retractor
A. lens forceps
A. lens hook
A. lip speculum
A. Mark II intraocular lens
A. needle holder
A. Tripod eye implant
A. tying forceps
A. utility forceps

B

Babcock
- B. Endo Grasp
- B. jointed vein stripper
- B. needle
- B. plate
- B. retractor
- B. stainless steel suture wire
- B. thoracic tissue forceps
- B. thoracic tissue-holding forceps
- B. tissue clamp
- B.-Beasley forceps

backbiter
- MicroFrance pediatric b.

BacFix system

Backhaus
- B. cervical knife
- B. dilator
- B. forceps
- B. towel clip

Baerveldt glaucoma implant

bag
- Bardex b.
- Bomgart stomal b.
- Brake hemostatic b.
- CLO Cool b.
- Endobag specimen b.
- Endopouch Pro specimen-retrieval b.
- Endosac specimen b.
- Endo-Sock b.
- Frenta enteral feeding b.
- Incono g.
- Karaya seal ileostomy stomal b.
- Lahey b.
- Ponsky Endo-Sock specimen retrieval b.
- Rusch leg b.
- Rutzen ileostomy g.
- Sones hemostatic b.
- Swenko b.

Baggish hysteroscope

Bahnson
- B. aortic aneurysm clamp
- B. aortic cannula
- B. appendage clamp
- B. sternal retractor

Baird chalazion forceps

BAK
- B. cage
- B. interbody fusion system
- B. laparoscopic procedure
- B./C cervical interbody fusion system
- B./Proximity interbody fusion implant

Baladi Inverter

Balfour
- B. bladder blade
- B. clamp
- B.

Balkin Up & Over introducer

balloon
- Acucise b.
- Ballobes gastric b.
- Bardex b.
- Bilisystem stone-removal b.
- Brandt cytology b.
- Cook b.
- Fogarty b.
- Giesy ureteral dilatation b.
- Grüntzig b.
- Honan b.
- Inoue self-guiding b.
- Monorail Speedy b.
- Origin b.
- Quantum TTC biliary b.
- QuickFurl b.
- RediFurl b.
- Rigiflex b.
- Sengstaken b.
- Short Speedy b.
- Stealth catheter b.

balloon (*continued*)
    TEGwire b.
    ThermaChoice uterine b.
    Xomed dual-chamber b.

band
    anchor b.
    Falope-ring tubal occlusion
      b.
    Flexi-Ty vessel b.
    Matas vessel b.
    Silastic b.
    Storz b.
    Watzke b.

bandage
    Champ elastic b.
    Comperm tubular b.
    E. Cotton b.
    Elastic Foam b.
    Elastomull b.
    Flexilite conforming elastic
      b.
    Fractura Flex b.
    Hydron Burn b.
    Liquiderm liquid healing b.
    Profore four-layer b.
    Tricodur Epi (elbow)
      compression support b.
    Tricodur Omos (shoulder)
      compression support b.
    Tricodur Talus (ankle)
      compression support b.
    Velpeau b.

Bankart tack

Bard
    B. Commander PTCA guide
      wire
    B. Composix mesh
    B. endoscopic suturing
      system (BESS)
    B. Memotherm colorectal
      stent
    B. PDA umbrella
    B. Sperma-Tex preshaped
      mesh
    B. TransAct intra-aortic
      balloon pump

Bard (*continued*)
    B. Visilex mesh
    B. XT coronary stent

BardPort implanted port

Barouk
    B. button
    B. cannulated bone screw
    B. microscrew
    B. microstaple

Barraquer
    B. Colibri forceps
    B. corneoscleral scissors
    B. iris scissors

barrier
    Capset bone graft b.
    Durahesive skin b.
    Interceed absorbable
      adhesion b.
    Marlen SkinShield adhesive
      skin b.
    Nu-Hope adhesive
      waterproof skin b.
    Oxiplex adhesive b.

bed
    Acucare b.
    Affinity b.
    Barikare b.
    Clini-Care b.
    Clini-Dyne b.
    Clini-Float b.
    Clinitron air b.
    Gatch b.
    KinAir b.
    Roho b.
    Skytron b.
    Stryker CircOlectric b.

beStent
    b. coronary stent
    b. Rival coronary stent
      system

Beta-Cath system

BiLAP
    B. bipolar cutting and
      coagulating prote

BiLAP (*continued*)
    B. bipolar needle electrode

Biobrane adhesive

BioCuff
    B. screw
    B. washer

BiodivYsio stent
    B. AS (added support) s.
    B. OC (open cell) s.
    B. SV (small vessel) s.

BioStinger bioabsorbable
  meniscal implant

blade
    Acra-Cut Spiral craniotome
      b.
    arachnoid-shape b.
    ASSI disposable cranio b.
    banana b.
    Beaver DeBakey b.
    Beaver keratome b.
    Castroviejo b.
    Cloward b.
    Cottle b.
    Curdy b.
    Dyonics disposable
      arthroscope b.
    Endo-Assist b.
    5-prong rake b.
    Franceschetti-type
      freeblade
    Fugo b.
    Goulian b.
    Grieshaber b.
    Hebra b.
    Hemostatix scalpel b.
    K-blade
    Kjelland b.
    LaForce b.
    LaserSonics EndoBlade
    Mako shaver b.
    Merlin bendable b.
    Meyerding retractor b.
    MVR b.
    Orca b.
    Paufique b.

blade (*continued*)
    RAD40 sinus b.
    sickle-shape b.
    Superblade
    Swann-Morton surgical b.
    Typhoon microdebrider b.
    Vascutech circular b.
    Yu-Holtgrewe malleable b.
    Zalkind-Balfour b.

Bogota bag

BONE-LOK bone fixation system

BonePlast bone void filler

Bookler swivel-ball laparoscopic
  instrument holder

Bookwalter retractor system

boot
    Cam walker b.
    Bunny b.
    Chukka b.
    Gelocast Unna b.
    Jobst b.
    Moon b.
    rocker b.
    Spenco b.
    Unna b.
    Venodyne b.
    Wilke b.

Bores
    B. corneal fixation forceps
    B. radial marker
    B. U-shaped forceps

bougie
    EndoLumina b.

Bowen wire tightener

Boyle uterine elevator

Boynton needle holder

brace
    Aircast Swivel-Strap b.
    Bledsoe b.
    Cast Boot hip abduction b.
    chair-back b.
    clamshell b.

brace (*continued*)
- CRS b. (Counter Rotation System)
- Cruiser hip abduction b.
- C. Ti. b.
- DonJoy Goldpoint knee b.
- 49er knee b.
- Friedman Splint b.
- gait lock splint b. (GLS)
- Galveston metacarpal b.
- Jewett b.
- Kicker Pavlik harness b.
- Liberty CMC thumb b.
- KS 5 ACL b.
- Kydex b.
- Lenox Hill b.
- Moon Boot b.
- Newport MC hip orthosis b.
- Nextep knee b.
- Palumbo knee b.
- Rhino Triangle b.
- Rolyan tibial fracture b.
- Seton hip b.
- SmartBrace b.
- SmartWrap elbow b.
- Swede-O-Universal b.
- Swivel-Strap b.
- TLSO b.
- Townsend knee b.
- UBC b. (University of British Columbia)

brace (*continued*)
- Ultrabrace
- Wheaton Pavlik harness b.

Branemark endosteal implant

Brent pressure earring

bronchoscope
- Chevalier Jackson b.
- Foroblique b.
- Fujinon flexible b.
- Holinger b.
- Holinger-Jackson b.
- Jackson b.
- Overhold-Jackson b.
- Safar b.
- Savary b.
- Shapshay laser b.
- Storz infant b.
- Xanar laser b.
- Yankauer b.

brush
- Geenan cytology b.

Bunnell
- B. hand and finger splints
- B. knuckle bender
- B. tendon stripper

Buselmeier shunt

Button-One Step gastrostomy device

C

Calandruccio triangular compression fixation device

calcar reamer

Calcitek
C. drill system
C. spline

Calcitite alloplastic bone replacement material

cannula
Abelson cricothyrotomy c.
Becker accelerator c.
DeRoyal c.
DirectFlow arterial c.
Embol-X arterial c.
Fluoro Tip c.
Grinfeld c.
Kanavel brain-exploring c.
Mladick c.
MultAport c.

Capio CL transvaginal suture-capturing device

CAPS ArthroWand

Cardiomed
C. Bodysoft epidural catheter
C. endotracheal ventilation catheter
C. thermodilation catheter

CardioSEAL septal occluder

cast
Aquaplast c.
Fractura Flex
Frejka c.
Gypsona
Hexcelite
MaxCast
Muenster c.
Neufeld c.
Orfizip knee c.
Orthoplast slipper c.
Risser-Cotrel body c.

cast (*continued*)
Ortho-Glass
Sarmiento

catheter
7F Hydrolyser thrombectomy c.
A1, A2 Port multipurpose c.
Abbokinase c.
Ablaser laser delivery c.
Abramson c.
ablation c.
Abscession biliary drainage c.
Achiever balloon dilatation c
ACMI Alcock c.
ACMI Bunts c.
ACMI coated Foley c.
ACMI Emmett hemostatic c.
ACMI Owens c.
ACMI positive pressure c.
ACMI severance c.
ACMI Thackston c.
ACMI ureteral c.
ACMI Word Bartholin gland c.
ACS Concorde dilatation c.
ACS Endura coronary dilatation c.
ACS OTW (over-the-wire) Lifestream coronary dilatation c.
ACS Tourguide II guiding c.
AcuNav diagnostic ultrasound c.
Acucise RP retrograde endopyelotomy c.
Adante PTCA balloon c.
AFocus c.
Ahn thrombectomy c.
Alert-TD c.
Alliance c.
Alzate c.
Amazr c.
Angiocath PRN c.

catheter (*continued*)

Anthron heparinized c.
Antibacterial personal c.
Arrowgard Blue Line c.
Arrow-Howes multilumen c.
Arrow TheraCath epidural c.
Arrow Twin Cath c.
Ascent guiding c.
AtheroCath c.
Atlantis SR coronary intravascular ultrasound c.
Auth atherectomy c.
BD Insyte Autoguard shielded intravenous c.
Bard Stinger S. ablation c.
Beta-Cath c.
bifoil balloon c.
Blue FlexTip c.
Brevi-Kath epidural c.
Bronchitrac L c.
Broviac c.
Burhenne steerable c.
Calypso Rely c.
Camino intracranial c.
Cardiac Assist intra-aortic balloon c.
Cardiomed Bodysoft epidural c.
Cardiomed endotracheal ventilation c.
Cardiomed thermodilution c.
Cardio Tactilaze peripheral angioplasty laser c.
Cheetah angioplasty c.
Chemo-Port c.
Chilli cooled ablation c.
CliniCath c.
Conceptus Soft Seal cervical c.
Conceptus Soft torque uterine c.
Conceptus VS c.
Constellation mapping c.
Cool Tip c.
Cordis Predator PTCA balloon c.

catheter (*continued*)

Cordis Trakstar PTCA balloon c.
coude c.
CrossSail coronary dilatation c.
CryoCath c.
Datascope c.
Desai VectorCath c.
Dobbhoff c.
Dorros infusion and probing c.
Du Pen c.
DURAglide stone balloon c.
EAC c.
EchoMark c.
Endotak C. lead c.
Endura dilatation c.
EnSite cardiac c.
Erythroflex c.
Evert-O-Cath
eXamine cholangiography c.
Express PTCA c.
Extreme laser c.
FACT c.
Falcon coronary c.
Feth-R-Kath epidural c.
Flexguard tip c.
Flexxicon c.
Flexxicon Blue c.
Flow Rider flow-directed c.
Focus -PV balloon c.
Force balloon dilatation c.
Fountain infusion c.
Freeway PTCA c
FullFlow perfusion dilation c.
Gazelle balloon dilatation c.
Gold Probe bipolar hemostasis c.
Grollman c.
Groshong c.
Grüntzig balloon c.
Guardian c.
GyneSys Dx diagnostic c.
Halo XP c.
Hassan c.

catheter (*continued*)
- HealthShield c.
- Hemo-Cath c.
- Hohn central venous c.
- Hurwitz dialysis c.
- Illumen-8 guiding c.
- Infiniti c.
- Innervision ventricular c.
- Insyte AutoGuard c.
- IVUS .
- Jocath Maestro coronary balloon c.
- Jography angiographic c.
- Joguide coronary guiding c.
- Kifia c.
- Kinsey atherectomy c.
- Konton c.
- latis dual-lumen graft-cleaning c.
- LeMaitre biliary c.
- Leonard c.
- LifeJet high-flow chronic dialysis c.
- Lifestream coronary dilatation c.
- Livewire Duo-Decapolar c.
- Livewire TC Compass ablation c.
- Lynx over-the-wire balloon c.
- Maverick balloon dilatation c.
- Max Force c.
- Medcomp c.
- MegaSonics PTCA c.
- Mercator c.
- MicroMewi multi-sidehole infusion c.
- Millenia balloon c.
- Monorail c.
- NavAblator c.
- Naviport hollow-lumen guiding c.
- NeuroEdge neurovascular c.
- NoProfile balloon c.
- Nutricath silicone elastomer c.

catheter (*continued*)
- OmniCath atherectomy c.
- On-Command c.
- OpenSail balloon c.
- Opticon c.
- Opti-Plast XT balloon c.
- OptiQue sensing c.
- Oracle MegaSonics coronary balloon/imaging c.
- Oreopoulos-Zellerman c.
- Pacel bipolar pacing c.
- Parahisian EP c.
- ParCA c.
- Parodi c.
- P.A.S. Port c.
- Passage c.
- PBN hysterosalpingography c.
- Periflow peripheral balloon c.
- Per-Q-Cath
- Phantom V Plus c.
- Pico-T II PTCA balloon c.
- Pipelle endometrial suction c.
- Pleurx pleural c
- Pollock c.
- PolyFlo peripherally inserted central c.
- Porterfield c.
- Powerflex balloon c.
- Point 9 c.
- ProCross Rely over-the-wire balloon c.
- Quinton Mahurkar dual lumen c.
- Racz epidural c.
- Ranfac cholangiographic c.
- Rebar microvascular c.
- Redifurl Taperseal c.
- Ref-Star EP c.
- Release-NF c.
- Rhyder diagnostic c.
- RITA ablation c.
- Rivas vascular c.
- R1 Rapid Exchange balloon c.

catheter (*continued*)
    Rsch-Uchida transjugular liver access needle-c.
    Sable PTCA balloon c.
    Shaldon c.
    Sherpa guiding c.
    Shone c.
    Simpson atherectomy c.
    Skinny dilatation c.
    Slinky c.
    Soaker c
    Soft Seal cervical c..
    Soft Torque uterine c.
    Solera thrombectomy c.
    SOS Omni c.
    Spectranetics support c.
    Spectrum silicone Foley c.
    SpineCATH c.
    Sprint c. with Pro/Pel coating
    Spyglass angiography c.
    Stamey-Malecot c.
    Stargate falloposcopy c.
    Suction Buster c.
    Supreme electrophysiology c.
    Surpass c.
    Syntel latex-free embolectomy c.
    Tactilaze angioplasty laser c.
    Takumi PTCA c.
    Talon balloon dilatation c.
    Telescope c.
    Tenckhoff peritoneal dialysis c.
    thermodilution c.
    Tis-u-trap endometrial suction c.
    Titan Mega PTCA dilatation c.
    Titan MEga XL PtCA dilatation c.
    Tourguide guiding c.
    Tracer over-the-wire intravascular mapping c.
    transluminal extraction c.
    TUN-L-KATH epidural c.

catheter (*continued*)
    TTS (through the scope) c.
    Uldall subclavian hemodialysis c.
    Ureflex ureteral c.
    UroMax II c.
    Vas-Cath c
    Vascu-Sheath c.
    Vector large-lumen c.
    Ventric True Tech ICP c.
    Veripath peripheral guiding c.
    Vitesse c.
    VNUS Restore v.
    Vueport balloon-occlusion c.
    Workhorse percutaneous transluminal angioplasty balloon c.
    Xpeedior 100 c.
    X-Sizer c.
    XXL balloon dilatation c.
    Z-Med c.
    Zuma guiding c.

cautery
    Aaron c.
    Acucise ureteral cutting c.
    BiLAP bipolar c.
    Concept handheld c.
    Endocut c. device
    Mira c.
    Neoknife c.
    Op-Temp c.

cavernotome

Cell Saver 5

cement
    BA bone c.
    BoneSource hydroxyapatite c.
    Endurance bone c.
    Simplex-P bone c.
    SRS injectable c.
    Terlux c.
    VersaBond c.

Cho/Dyonics two-portal endoscopic system

choledochofiberscope

Chonstruct chondral repair system

Christoudias fascial wound closure device

Chronicle implantable hemodynamic monitor

Ciaglia percutaneous tracheostomy introducer

CircAid elastic stockings

Circon videohydrothoracoscope

CirKuit-Guard device

clamp
    Abadie enterostomy c.
    Ablaza patent ductus c.
    Abramson-Allis breast c.
    Acland microvascular c.
    Adair breast c.
    Adson c.
    Adson-Brown c.
    agraffe c.
    Ahlquist-Durham embolism c.
    Alfred M. Large vena cava c.
    Allen anastomosis c.
    Allen intestinal c.
    Allen-Kocher c.
    Allis tissue c.
    Allison c.
    Alyea vas c.
    anastomosis c.
    Ando aortic c.
    aneurysm c.
    angled DeBakey c.
    angled peripheral vascular c.
    Ann Arbor towel c.
    anterior resection c.
    aortic aneurysm c.
    aortic cannula c.
    aortic occlusion c.
    appendage c.
    arterial c.

clamp (*continued*)
    Asch c.
    ASSI METE-5168 Microspike approximator c.
    ASSI METS-3668 Microspike approximator c.
    ASSI MKCV-2040 Microspike approximator c.
    ASSI MSPK-3678 Microspike approximator c.
    Atlee bronchus c.
    Atra-Grip c.
    atraumatic intestinal c.
    Atraumax peripheral vascular c.
    atrial c.
    Ault intestinal c.
    auricular appendage c.
    Auvard c.
    Babcock tissue c.
    baby Bishop c.
    baby Kocher c.
    baby pylorus c.
    baby Satinsky c.
    Backhaus towel c.
    Backhaus-Jones towel c.
    Backhaus-Kocher towel c.
    Bahnson aortic aneurysm c.
    Bahnson appendage c.
    Bailey aortic c.
    Bailey duckbill c.
    Bailey-Cowley c.
    Bailey-Morse c.
    Bainbridge anastomosis c.
    Bainbridge intestinal c.
    Bainbridge vessel c.
    Balfour c.
    Ballantine c.
    Bamby c.
    bar-to-bar c.
    Bard Cunningham incontinence c.
    Barraquer needle holder c.
    Bartley anastomosis c.
    Bartley partial-occlusion c.
    Bauer kidney pedicle c.
    Baumrucker post-TUR irrigation c.

clamp (*continued*)

Baumrucker urinary incontinence c.
Baumrucker-DeBakey c.
Beall bulldog c.
Beall-Morris ascending aortic c.
Beardsley intestinal c.
Beck aortic c.
Beck vascular c.
Beck vessel c.
Beck-Potts aortic c.
Beck-Potts pulmonic c.
Beck-Satinsky c.
Belcher c.
Benson pyloric c.
Berens muscle c.
Berke c.
Berke ptosis c.
Berkeley c.
Berkeley-Bonney vaginal c.
Berman aortic c.
Berman vascular c.
Bernhard c.
Berry pile c.
Best intestinal c.
Bethune c.
Bielawski heart c.
Bigelow calvaria c.
Bihrle dorsal c.
Bircher bone-holding c.
Bircher cartilage c.
Bishop bone c.
Black meatal c.
Blair cleft palate c.
Blalock pulmonary artery c.
Blalock-Niedner pulmonic stenosis c.
Blanchard pile c.
Blasucci c.
blepharostat c.
bloodless circumcision c.
Boettcher pulmonary artery c.
Böhler os calcis c.
bone extension c.
bone-holding c.
Bonney c.

clamp (*continued*)

Borge bile duct c.
Bortz c.
Boyes muscle c.
Bozeman c.
Bradshaw-O'Neill aortic c.
Bridge c.
Brock auricular c.
Brockington pile c.
Brodney urethrographic c.
Bronner c.
Brown lip c.
Brunner colon c.
Brunner intestinal c.
Buie pile c.
Buie-Hirschman pile c.
bulldog c.
Bunke c.
Bunnell-Howard arthrodesis c.
Burford c.
Burlisher c.
Bushey compression c.
Buxton uterine c.
C-c.
Cairns c.
Calandruccio c.
Calman carotid c.
Calman ring c.
calvarial c.
cannula c.
Capes c.
Cardio-Grip anastomosis c.
Cardio-Grip aortic c.
Cardio-Grip bronchus c.
Cardio-Grip pediatric c.
Cardio-Grip renal artery c.
Cardio-Grip tangential occlusion c.
Cardio-Grip vascular c.
cardiovascular anastomotic c.
cardiovascular bulldog c.
Carmalt c.
Carmel c.
carotid artery c.
Carrel c.
clamp carrier

clamp (*continued*)
    Carter c.
    Carter-Glassman resection
      c.
    cartilage c.
    caruncle c.
    Casey pelvic c.
    Castaneda anastomosis c.
    Castaneda IMM vascular c.
    Castaneda partial-occlusion
      c.
    Castaneda vascular c.
    Castaneda-Mixter thoracic
      c.
    Castroviejo lens c.
    Castroviejo mosquito lid c.
    Castroviejo needle holder c.
    cautery c.
    caval occlusion c.
    celiac c.
    cervical c.
    chalazion c.
    Charnley arthrodesis c.
    Charnley bone c.
    Charnley external fixation c.
    Charnley pin c.
    cholangiography c.
    circumcision c.
    Clairborne c.
    Clevis c.
    cloth-shod c.
    coarctation c.
    Codman cartilage c.
    Codman towel c.
    Collier thoracic c.
    Collin umbilical c.
    colon c.
    colostomy c.
    columellar c.
    Conger perineal
      urethrostomy c.
    contour block c.
    Cooley acutely-curved c.
    Cooley anastomosis c.
    Cooley aortic aneurysm c.
    Cooley aortic cannula c.
    Cooley bronchial c.
    Cooley bulldog c.

clamp (*continued*)
    Cooley carotid c.
    Cooley caval occlusion c.
    Cooley coarctation c.
    Cooley cross-action bulldog
      c.
    Cooley curved
      cardiovascular c.
    Cooley double-angled c.
    Cooley graft c.
    Cooley iliac c.
    Cooley neonatal vascular c.
    Cooley partial-occlusion c.
    Cooley patent ductus c.
    Cooley pediatric vascular c.
    Cooley peripheral vascular
      c.
    Cooley renal artery c.
    Cooley subclavian c.
    Cooley tangential pediatric
      c.
    Cooley vena cava c.
    Cooley-Baumgarten aortic
      c.
    Cooley-Beck vessel c.
    Cooley-Derra anastomosis
      c.
    Cooley-Satinsky c.
    Cope crushing c.
    Cope modification of Martel
      intestinal c.
    Cope-DeMartel c.
    cordotomy c.
    Cottle columellar c.
    cotton-roll rubber-dam c.
    Crafoord aortic c.
    Crafoord auricular c.
    Crafoord coarctation c.
    Crafoord-Sellors auricular c.
    Crenshaw caruncle c.
    Crile appendiceal c.
    Crile crushing c.
    Crile hemostatic c.
    Crile-Crutchfield c.
    Cross c.
    cross-action bulldog c.
    cross-action towel c.
    Cruickshank entropion c.

clamp (*continued*)
  crushing c.
  Crutchfield carotid artery c.
  Cunningham urinary
    incontinence c.
  curved cardiovascular c.
  curved Mayo c.
  curved mosquito c.
  curved-8 c.
  Cushing c.
  cystic duct catheter c.
  D'Allesandro c.
  D'Assumpcão c.
  Dacron graft c.
  Daems bronchial c.
  Dandy c.
  Daniel colostomy c.
  Dardik c.
  David-Baker lip c.
  Davidson muscle c.
  Davidson pulmonary vessel
    c.
  Davila atrial c.
  Davis aortic aneurysm c.
  Dean MacDonald gastric
    resection c.
  Deaver c.
  DeBakey aortic aneurysm c.
  DeBakey aortic exclusion c.
  DeBakey arterial c.
  DeBakey bulldog c.
  DeBakey coarctation c.
  DeBakey cross-action
    bulldog c.
  DeBakey curved peripheral
    vascular c.
  DeBakey patent ductus c.
  DeBakey pediatric c.
  DeBakey peripheral
    vascular c.
  DeBakey ring-handled
    bulldog c.
  DeBakey S-shaped
    peripheral vascular c.
  DeBakey tangential
    occlusion c.
  DeBakey-Bahnson vascular
    c.

clamp (*continued*)
  DeBakey-Bainbridge
    vascular c.
  DeBakey-Beck c.
  DeBakey-Crafoord vascular
    c.
  DeBakey-Derra
    anastomosis c.
  DeBakey-Harken auricular
    c.
  DeBakey-Howard aortic
    aneurysm c.
  DeBakey-Kay aortic c.
  DeBakey-McQuigg-Mixter
    bronchial c.
  DeBakey-Satinsky vena
    cava c.
  DeBakey-Semb c.
  DeCourcy goiter c.
  DeMartel vascular c.
  DeMartel-Wolfson
    anastomosis c.
  DeMartel-Wolfson colon c.
  DeMartel-Wolfson intestinal
    c.
  Demel wire c.
  Demos tibial artery c.
  Dennis anastomotic c.
  Dennis intestinal c.
  Derra anastomosis c.
  Derra aortic c.
  Derra vena cava c.
  Derra vestibular c.
  Desmarres lid c.
  Devonshire-Mack c.
  DeWeese vena cava c.
  Dick bronchus c.
  Dick pressure c.
  Dieffenbach bulldog c.
  Diethrich aortic c.
  Diethrich graft c.
  Diethrich microcoronary
    bulldog c.
  Diethrich shunt c.
  Dingman cartilage c.
  disposable muscle biopsy
    c.
  dissecting c.

clamp (*continued*)
- distraction c.
- Dixon-Thomas-Smith intestinal c.
- Dobbie-Trout bulldog c.
- Doctor Collins fracture c.
- Doctor Long c.
- Dogliotti-Gugliel mini c.
- Dolphin cord c.
- Donald c.
- double Softjaw c.
- double towel c.
- double-angled c.
- Downing c.
- Doyen intestinal c.
- Doyen towel c.
- drape c.
- dreamer c.
- duckbill c.
- ductus c.
- duodenal c.
- Duval lung c.
- Earle hemorrhoidal c.
- C. Ease device
- Eastman intestinal c.
- Edebohls kidney c.
- Edna towel c.
- Edwards double Softjaw c.
- Edwards single Softjaw c.
- Edwards spring c.
- Efteklar c.
- Eisenstein c.
- endoaortic c.
- English c.
- enterostomy c.
- entropion c.
- Erhardt lid c.
- Ericksson-Stille carotid c.
- Ewald-Hudson c.
- Ewing lid c.
- exclusion c.
- extension bone c.
- extracutaneous vas fixation c.
- Falk c.
- Farabeuf bone c.
- Farabeuf-Lambotte bone-holding c.

clamp (*continued*)
- Fauer peritoneal c.
- Favaloro proximal anastomosis c.
- Favorite c.
- feather c.
- Fehland intestinal c.
- Fehland right-angled colon c.
- femoral c.
- Ferguson bone c.
- Ferrier 212 gingival c.
- ferrule c.
- fine-tooth c.
- Finochietto arterial c.
- Finochietto bronchial c.
- Fitzgerald aortic aneurysm c.
- flexible aortic c.
- flexible retractor pressure c.
- flexible retractor sliding c.
- flexible vascular c.
- flow-regulator c.
- Fogarty Hydragrip c.
- Fogarty-Chin c.
- c. forceps
- Ford c.
- Forrester c.
- Foss anterior resection c.
- Foss cardiovascular c.
- Foss intestinal c.
- Frahur cartilage c.
- Frazier-Adson osteoplastic c.
- Frazier-Sachs c.
- Freeman c.
- Friedrich c.
- Friedrich-Petz c.
- Fukushima C-clamp c.
- full-curved c.
- Furness anastomosis c.
- Furness-Clute anastomosis c.
- Furness-Clute duodenal c.
- Furness-McClure-Hinton c.
- gallbladder ring c.
- Gam-Mer aneurysm c.
- Gam-Mer occlusion c.

clamp (*continued*)
    Gandy c.
    Gant c.
    Garcia aorta c.
    Garcia aortic c.
    Gardner skull c.
    Garland hysterectomy c.
    Gaskell c.
    gastric c.
    gastroenterostomy c.
    gastrointestinal c.
    Gavin-Miller c.
    Gemini c.
    Gerald c.
    Gerbode patent ductus c.
    Gerster bone c.
    GI c.
    gingival c.
    Gladstone-Putterman
        transmarginal rotation
        entropion c.
    Glass liver-holding c.
    Glassman bowel atraumatic
        c.
    Glassman intestinal c.
    Glassman liver-holding c.
    Glassman noncrushing
        gastroenterostomy c.
    Glassman noncrushing
        gastrointestinal c.
    Glassman-Allis c.
    Glover auricular c.
    Glover auricular-appendage
        c.
    Glover bulldog c.
    Glover coarctation c.
    Glover curved c.
    Glover patent ductus c.
    Glover spoon-shaped
        anastomosis c.
    Glover vascular c.
    Glover-DeBakey c.
    Glover-Stille c.
    goiter c.
    Goldblatt c.
    Goldstein Microspike
        approximator c.
    Goldvasser c.

clamp (*continued*)
    Gomco bell c.
    Gomco bloodless
        circumcision c.
    Gomco umbilical cord c.
    Goodwin bone c.
    Grafco incontinence c.
    Grafco umbilical cord c.
    graft c.
    Grant aortic aneurysm c.
    grasping c.
    Gray c.
    Green bulldog c.
    Green lid c.
    Green suction tube-holding
        c.
    Greenberg c.
    Gregory baby profunda c.
    Gregory carotid bulldog c.
    Gregory external c.
    Gregory stay suture c.
    Gregory vascular miniature
        c.
    Gross coarctation c.
    Grover Atra-grip c.
    Grover auricular appendage
        c.
    Gusberg hysterectomy c.
    Gussenbauer c.
    gut c.
    Gutgemann auricular
        appendage c.
    Guyon kidney c.
    Guyon vessel c.
    Guyon-Péan vessel c.
    Haberer intestinal c.
    half-curved c.
    Halifax interlaminar c.
    Halsted curved mosquito c.
    Halsted straight mosquito c.
    handleless c.
    Harken auricular c.
    Harrah lung c.
    Harrington hook c.
    Harrington-Carmalt c.
    Harrington-Mixter thoracic
        c.
    Hartmann c.

clamp (*continued*)
   Harvey Stone c.
   Hatch c.
   Hausmann vascular c.
   Haverhill c.
   Haverhill-Mack c.
   Hayes anterior resection c.
   Hayes colon c.
   Hayes intestinal c.
   Heaney c.
   Heartport endoaortic c.
   Heifitz cerebral aneurysm c.
   Heitz-Boyer c.
   Hemoclip c.
   hemorrhoidal c.
   hemostatic c.
   Hendren cardiovascular c.
   Hendren ductus c.
   Hendren megaureter c.
   Hendren ureteral c.
   Henley subclavian artery c.
   Henley vascular c.
   Herbert Adams coarctation
      c.
   Herff c.
   Herrick kidney c.
   Herrick pedicle c.
   Hesseltine umbilical cord c.
   Hex-Fix Universal swivel c.
   Heyer-Schulte Rayport
      muscle biopsy c.
   Hibbs c.
   hilar c.
   Hirsch mucosal c.
   Hirschman pile c.
   Hoff towel c.
   Hoffmann ligament c.
   Hohmann c.
   c. holder
   Hollister c.
   Holter pump c.
   Hopener c.
   Hopkins aortic occlusion c.
   Hopkins hysterectomy c.
   Howard-DeBakey aortic
      aneurysm c.
   Hudson c.
   Hufnagel aortic c.

clamp (*continued*)
   Hume aortic c.
   Humphries aortic aneurysm
      c.
   Humphries reverse-curve
      aortic c.
   Hunt colostomy c.
   Hunter-Satinsky c.
   Hurson flexible
      pressure c.
   Hurson flexible sliding c.
   Hurwitz esophageal c.
   Hurwitz intestinal c.
   Hymes meatal c.
   hysterectomy c.
   iliac c.
   Iliff c.
   incontinence c.
   c. insert
   interlaminar c.
   intestinal anastomosis c.
   intestinal occlusion c.
   intestinal resection c.
   intestinal ring c.
   isoelastic rip c.
   Ivory rubber dam c.
   Jackson bone c.
   Jackson bone-extension c.
   Jackson bone-holding c.
   Jacobs c.
   Jacobson bulldog c.
   Jacobson microbulldog c.
   Jacobson vessel c.
   Jacobson-Potts vessel c.
   Jahnke anastomosis c.
   Jahnke-Cook-Seeley c.
   Jako c.
   Jameson muscle c.
   Jansen c.
   Jarit anterior resection c.
   Jarit cartilage c.
   Jarit intestinal c.
   Jarit meniscal c.
   Jarvis pile c.
   Javid bypass c.
   Javid carotid c.
   Jesberg laryngectomy c.
   Johns Hopkins bulldog c.

clamp (*continued*)
    Johns Hopkins coarctation
      c.
    Johns Hopkins modified
      Potts c.
    Johnston c.
    Jones thoracic c.
    Jones towel c.
    Joseph septal c.
    Judd c.
    Judd-Allis c.
    Juevenelle c.
    Julian-Damian c.
    Julian-Fildes c.
    K-Gar umbilical c.
    Kalt needle holder c.
    Kane obstetrical c.
    Kane umbilical cord c.
    Kantor circumcision c.
    Kantrowitz hemostatic c.
    Kantrowitz thoracic c.
    Kapp microarterial c.
    Kapp-Beck bronchial c.
    Kapp-Beck coarctation c.
    Kapp-Beck colon c.
    Kapp-Beck-Thomson c.
    Karamar-Mailatt
      tarsorhaphy c.
    Kartchner carotid artery c.
    Kaufman kidney c.
    Kay aortic anastomosis c.
    Kay-Lambert c.
    Kelly c.
    Kelsey pile c.
    Kern bone-holding c.
    Kersting colostomy c.
    Khan-Jaeger c.
    Khodadad c.
    kidney pedicle c.
    Kiefer c.
    Kindt arterial c.
    Kindt carotid c.
    King c.
    Kinsella-Buie lung c.
    Kitner c.
    Kleinert-Kutz c.
    Kleinschmidt
      appendectomy c.

clamp (*continued*)
    Klevas c.
    Klinikum-Berlin tubing c.
    Klintmalm c.
    Klute c.
    Knutsson penile c.
    Knutsson urethrography c.
    Kocher intestinal c.
    Kolodny c.
    Krosnick vesicourethral
      suspension c.
    Kutzmann c.
    Ladd lid c.
    Lahey bronchial c.
    Lahey thoracic c.
    Lalonde bone c.
    Lambert aortic c.
    Lambert-Kay aortic c.
    Lambert-Kay vascular c.
    Lambert-Lowman bone c.
    Lambotte bone-holding c.
    Lamis patellar c.
    c. lamp
    Lane bone-holding c.
    Lane gastroenterostomy c.
    Lane intestinal c.
    Lane towel c.
    laparoscopic Allis c.
    Large vena cava c. (Alfred
      M. Large)
    laryngectomy c.
    LCC lung compression c.
    Leahey c.
    Lee bronchus c.
    Lee microvascular c.
    Lees vascular c.
    Lees wedge resection c.
    Leland-Jones vascular c.
    Lem-Blay circumcision c.
    Lewin bone-holding c.
    lid c.
    Liddle aortic c.
    Life-Lok c.
    ligament c.
    Lillie rectus tendon c.
    Lin c.
    Lindner anastomosis c.
    Linnartz intestinal c.

clamp (*continued*)
  Linnartz stomach c.
  Linton tourniquet c.
  lion-head c.
  lion-jaw c.
  lip c.
  Litwak c.
  liver-holding c.
  Lloyd-Davies c.
  lobster-type c.
  Locke bone c.
  locking c.
  Lockwood c.
  Longmire-Storm c.
  Lorna nonperforating towel c.
  Lowman bone-holding c.
  Lowman-Gerster bone c.
  Lowman-Hoglund c.
  Lulu c.
  lung exclusion c.
  McCleery-Miller intestinal anastomosis c.
  McCullough hysterectomy c.
  McDonald gastric c.
  McDougal prostatectomy c.s
  McGuire c.
  McKenzie c.
  McLean c.
  McNealey-Glassman c.
  McNealey-Glassman-Mixter c.
  Madden intestinal c.
  Maingot c.
  Malgaigne c.
  Malis hinge c.
  Marcuse tube c.
  marginal c.
  Martel intestinal c.
  Martin cartilage c.
  Martin muscle c.
  Mason vascular c.
  Masters intestinal c.
  Masters-Schwartz intestinal c.
  Masters-Schwartz liver c.

clamp (*continued*)
  Masterson pelvic c.
  Mastin muscle c.
  Matthew cross-leg c.
  Mattox aortic c.
  May kidney c.
  Mayfield aneurysm c.
  Mayfield head c.
  Mayfield three-pin skull c.
  Mayo kidney c.
  Mayo vessel c.
  Mayo-Guyon kidney c.
  Mayo-Guyon vessel c.
  Mayo-Lovelace spur crushing c.
  Mayo-Robson intestinal c.
  McQuigg c.
  meatal c.
  Meeker gallstone c.
  Meeker right-angle c.
  megaureter c.
  meniscal c.
  Michel aortic c.
  microarterial c.
  microbulldog c.
  Microspike approximator c.
  microvascular c.
  Mikulicz peritoneal c.
  Mikulicz-Radecki c.
  Miles rectal c.
  Millard c.
  Millin c.
  miniature bulldog c.
  Mitchel aortotomy c.
  Mitchel-Adam c.
  Mixter ligature-carrier c.
  Mixter thoracic c.
  Mogen circumcision c.
  Mohr pinchcock c.
  Moreno gastroenterostomy c.
  Moria-France dacryocystorhinostomy c.
  Morris aortic c.
  mosquito hemostatic c.
  mosquito lid c.
  mouse-tooth c.
  Moynihan towel c.

clamp (*continued*)
Mueller aortic c.
Mueller bronchial c.
Mueller pediatric c.
Mueller vena cava c.
Muir rectal cautery c.
Mulligan anastomosis c.
multipurpose c.
muscle biopsy c.
mush c.
Myles hemorrhoidal c.
myocardial c.
Nakayama c.
Naraghi-DeCoster reduction c.
needle holder c.
neonatal vascular c.
nephrostomy c.
nerve-approximating c.
Nichols aortic c.
Nicola tendon c.
Niedner anastomosis c.
Niedner pulmonic c.
noncrushing anterior resection c.
noncrushing bowel c.
noncrushing gastroenterostomy c.
noncrushing gastrointestinal c.
noncrushing intestinal c.
noncrushing liver-holding c.
noncrushing vascular c.
nonperforating towel c.
Noon AV fistular c.
Nunez aortic c.
Nunez auricular c.
Nussbaum intestinal c.
O'Connor lid c.
occluding c.
Ochsner aortic c.
Ochsner arterial c.
Ochsner thoracic c.
Ockerblad kidney c.
Ockerblad vessel c.
O'Hanlon intestinal c.
Olivecrona aneurysm c.
Olsen cholangiogram c.

clamp (*continued*)
Omed bulldog vascular c.
O'Neill cardiac c.
O'Shaughnessy c.
ossicle-holding c.
osteoplastic flap c.
padded c.
parametrium c.
Parham-Martin bone-holding c.
Parker c.
Parker-Kerr intestinal c.
Parsonnet aortic c.
partial-occlusion c.
Partipilo c.
patellar cement c.
patent ductus c.
Payr gastrointestinal c.
Payr pylorus c.
Payr resection c.
Payr stomach c.
Péan hemostatic c.
Péan hysterectomy c.
Péan intestinal c.
Péan vessel c.
pediatric bulldog c.
pedicle c.
Peers towel c.
pelvic c.
Pemberton sigmoid c.
Pemberton spur-crushing c.
penile c.
Pennington c.
Percy c.
pericortical c.
peripheral vascular c.
peritoneal c.
phalangeal c.
Phaneuf c.
phantom c.
Phillips rectal c.
pile c.
Pilling microanastomosis c.
Pilling pediatric c.
pin-to-bar c.
pinchcock c.
placental c.
Plastibell circumcision c.

clamp (*continued*)
- point-of-reduction c.
- Pomeranz aortic c.
- Poppen aortic c.
- Poppen-Blalock carotid artery c.
- Poppen-Blalock-Salibi carotid c.
- post-TUR irrigation c.
- Potts aortic c.
- Potts cardiovascular c.
- Potts coarctation c.
- Potts divisional c.
- Potts patent ductus c.
- Potts pulmonic c.
- Potts-DeBakey c.
- Potts-Niedner aortic c.
- Potts-Satinsky c.
- Potts-Smith aortic c.
- Potts-Smith pulmonic c.
- Poutasse renal artery c.
- Presbyterian Hospital occluding c.
- Presbyterian Hospital T-c.
- Presbyterian Hospital tubing c.
- Preshaw c.
- Price muscle c.
- Price-Thomas bronchial c.
- Prince muscle c.
- Pringle c.
- Providence Hospital c.
- ptosis c.
- Pudenz-Heyer c.
- pulmonary arterial c.
- pulmonary embolism c.
- pulmonary nodulectomy c.
- pulmonary vessel c.
- pulmonic stenosis c.
- Putterman levator resection c.
- Putterman ptosis c.
- pylorus c.
- Quick Bend flex c.
- R-N c.
- Ralks thoracic c.
- Ramstedt c.
- Ranieri c.

clamp (*continued*)
- Rankin anastomosis c.
- Rankin intestinal c.
- Rankin stomach c.
- Ranzewski intestinal c.
- ratchet c.
- Ravich c.
- Rayport muscle c.
- reamer c.
- rectal c.
- Redo intestinal c.
- Reich-Nechtow arterial c.
- Reinhoff swan neck c.
- renal artery c.
- renal pedicle c.
- resection c.
- Reul aortic c.
- reverse-curve c.
- Reynolds dissecting c.
- Reynolds resection c.
- Reynolds vascular c.
- Rhinelander c.
- Rica arterial c.
- Rica microarterial c.
- Rica stem c.
- Rica vessel c.
- Richards bone c.
- right-angle colon c.
- ring c.
- ring-handled bulldog c.
- ring-jawed holding c.
- Robin chalazion c.
- Rochester hook c.
- Rochester sigmoid c.
- Rochester-Kocher c.
- Rochester-Péan c.
- Rockey vascular c.
- Roe aortic tourniquet c.
- Roeder towel c.
- Roosen c.
- Roosevelt gastroenterostomy c.
- Roosevelt gastrointestinal c.
- root rubber dam c.
- rubber shod c.
- rubber-dam c.
- Rubin bronchial c.
- Rubio wire-holding c.

clamp (*continued*)
    Rubovits c.
    Rumel myocardial c.
    Rumel rubber c.
    Rumel thoracic c.
    Rush bone c.
    S-shaped peripheral
        vascular c.
    S. S. White c.
    Salibi carotid artery c.
    Santulli c.
    Sarnoff aortic c.
    Sarot arterial c.
    Sarot bronchus c.
    Satinsky anastomosis c.
    Satinsky aortic c.
    Satinsky pediatric c.
    Satinsky vascular c.
    Satinsky vena cava c.
    Schaedel cross-action towel
        c.
    Schlein c.
    Schlesinger c.
    Schnidt c.
    Schoemaker intestinal c.
    Schumacher aortic c.
    Schutz c.
    Schwartz arterial aneurysm
        c.
    Schwartz bulldog c.
    Schwartz intracranial c.
    Schwartz vascular c.
    Scoville-Lewis c.
    screw occlusive c.
    Scudder intestinal c.
    Scudder stomach c.
    Sehrt c.
    Seidel bone-holding c.
    Sellor c.
    Selman c.
    Selverstone carotid artery c.
    Semb bone-holding c.
    Semb bronchus c.
    Senning featherweight
        bulldog c.
    Senning-Stille c.
    septal c.
    serrefine c.

clamp (*continued*)
    Sheehy ossicle-holding c.
    Sheldon c.
    shutoff c.
    side-biting c.
    sidewinder aortic c.
    Siegler-Hellman c.
    sigmoid anastomosis c.
    Silber microvascular c.
    Silber vasovasostomy c.
    Sims-Maier c.
    Singley intestinal c.
    Siniscal eyelid c.
    skull c.
    Slim Fit flex c.
    Slocum meniscal c.
    slotted nerve c.
    SMIC intestinal c.
    Smith bone c.
    Smith cordotomy c.
    Smith marginal c.
    Smithwick anastomotic c.
    Softjaw c.
    Somers uterine c.
    Southwick c.
    sponge c.
    spoon anastomosis c.
    spur-crushing c.
    St. Mark c.
    St. Vincent tube c.
    stainless steel c.
    Stallard head c.
    Stanton cautery c.
    Stay-Rite c.
    Stayce adjustable c.
    Steinhauser bone c.
    Stemp c.
    stenosis c.
    Stepita meatal c.
    Stetten intestinal c.
    Stevenson c.
    Stille kidney c.
    Stille vessel c.
    Stille-Crawford coarctation
        c.
    Stimson pedicle c.
    Stiwer towel c.
    Stockman meatal c.

clamp (*continued*)
Stockman penile c.
stomach c.
Stone intestinal c.
Stone stomach c.
Stone-Holcombe
   anastomosis c.
Stone-Holcombe intestinal c.
Stony splenorenal shunt c.
Storey c.
Storz meatal c.
straight mosquito c.
Stratte kidney c.
Strauss meatal c.
Strauss penile c.
Strauss-Valentine penile c.
Strelinger colon c.
Subramanian classic
   miniature aortic c.
Subramanian sidewinder
   aortic c.
Sugarbaker retrocolic c.
Sugita head c.
Sumner c.
SurgiMed c.
Swan aortic c.
swan-neck c.
Swenson ring-jawed
   holding c.
Swiss bulldog c.
Sztehlo umbilical c.
T c.
tangential occlusion c.
tangential pediatric c.
Tatum meatal c.
Taufic cholangiography c.
Tehl c.
temporalis transfer c.
tension c.
Textor vasectomy c.
Thoma c.
Thompson carotid artery c.
Thomson lung c.
thoracic c.
Thorlakson lower occlusive
   c.
Thorlakson upper occlusive
   c.

clamp (*continued*)
three-bladed c.
Thumb-Saver introducer c.
tissue occlusion c.
tonsil c.
tonsillar c.
towel c.
Trendelenburg-Crafoord
   coarctation c.
Treves intestinal c.
trochanter-holding c.
truncus c.
Trusler infant vascular c.
tube-occluding c.
tubing c.
Tucker appendix c.
turkey-claw c.
Tydings tonsillar c.
Tyrrell c.
Ullrich tubing c.
Ulrich bone-holding c.
umbilical cord c.
Umbilicutter c.
Universal wire c.
upper occlusive c.
ureteral c.
urethrographic cannula c.
urinary incontinence c.
uterine c.
vaginal cuff c.
Valdoni c.
Vanderbilt vessel c.
Varco dissecting c.
Varco gallbladder c.
vas c.
Vasconcelos-Barretto c.
VascuClamp minibulldog
   vessel c.
VascuClamp vascular c.
vascular graft c.
vasovasostomy c.
Veidenheimer resection c.
vena cava c.
Verbrugge bone c.
Verbrugge bone-holding c.
Verse-Webster c.
vessel c.
vessel-occluding c.

clamp (*continued*)
  vestibular c.
  Virtus splinter c.
  von Petz intestinal c.
  Vorse tube-occluding c.
  Vorse-Webster tube-
    occluding c.
  vulsellum c.
  Wadsworth lid c.
  Walther kidney pedicle c.
  Walther pedicle c.
  Walther-Crenshaw meatal
    c.
  Walton meniscal c.
  Wangensteen anastomosis
    c.
  Wangensteen gastric-
    crushing anastomotic c.
  Wangensteen patent
    ductus c.
  Warthen spur-crushing c.
  Watts locking c.
  Weaver chalazion c.
  Weber aortic c.
  Weck c.
  Weck-Edna nonperforating
    towel c.
  wedge resection c.
  Weldon miniature bulldog
    c.
  Wells pedicle c.
  Wertheim kidney pedicle c.
  Wertheim-Cullen kidney
    pedicle c.
  Wertheim-Reverdin pedicle
    c.
  West Shur cartilage c.
  Wester meniscal c.
  White c.
  Whitver penile c.
  Wikström gallbladder c.
  Wikström-Stilgust c.
  Willett c.
  Williams c.
  Wilman c.
  Wilson c.
  Winkelmann circumcision
    c.

clamp (*continued*)
  Winston cervical c.
  wire-tightening c.
  Wirthlin splenorenal shunt
    c.
  Wister vascular c.
  Wolfson intestinal c.
  Wolfson spur-crushing c.
  Wood bulldog c.
  Wylie carotid artery c.
  Wylie hypogastric c.
  Wylie lumbar bulldog c.
  X-c.
  Yasargil carotid c.
  Yellen circumcision c.
  Young renal pedicle c.
  Z-c.
  Zachary-Cope c.
  Zachary-Cope-DeMartel
    colon c.
  Zeppelin c.
  Ziegler-Furness c.
  Zimmer cartilage c.
  Zinnanti c.
  Zipser meatal c.
  Zipser penile c.
  Zutt c.
  Zweifel appendectomy c.
  Zweifel pressure c.

clamshell
  c. brace
  c. incision

Clarion
  C. CII Bionic Ear system
  C. CII BTE (behind the ear)
    sound processor
  C. cochlear implant
  C. HiFocus electrode
  C. multi-strategy cochlear
    implant
  C. Platinum BTE sound
    processor

Clarus spinescope

cleansers
  Biolex c.
  CarraKleenz c.

cleansers (*continued*)
    Carrington c.
    Clinswound c.
    Dey-Wash skin wound c.
    DiabKlenz wound c.
    Hibiclens c.
    Hibistat c.
    Hibitane c.
    Prepodyne solution
    Septicare c.
    Sklar c.
    UltraKlenz wound c.

ClearCut 2 electrosurgical handpiece

clip
    Autostat hemostatic c.
    Endo GIA surgical c.
    Filshie female sterilization c.
    Hegenbarth c.
    Hemoclip c.
    Hem-o-lok c.
    Hesseltine Umbili c.
    Hulka c.
    Hulka-Clemens c.
    MicroMark c.
    Perneczky aneurysm c.
    Rica suture c.
    Schwasser microclip c.
    Secu c.

CloseSure procedure kit

CO2 Heart Laser 2

coblation-based disposable arthroscopic

Codere orbital floor implant

Cofield total shoulder system

Coherent
    C. CO_2 laser
    C. UltraPulse 5000C laser
    C. Versapulse device

Cohn cardiac stabilizer

collagen hemostatic material
    Avitene

collagen hemostatic (*continued*)
    Bio-Oss
    bucrylate
    Collastat
    Contigen Bard
    Contigen glutaraldehyde
    Contigen implant
    Endo-Avitene
    Hemaflex sheath
    Helitene
    Hemopad
    Hemotene
    InterGard knitted.
    Instat
    Surgical Nu-Knit
    Surgicel
    Unilab Surgibone
    Zyclast
    Zyderm I or II

Collagraft bone graft matrix

Compliant pre-stress bone implant system

Conceptus
    C. Robust guide wire
    C. Soft Seal cervical catheter
    C. Soft Torque uterine catheter
    C. VS (variable softness) catheter

Concise compression hip screw system

Coopervision irrigation/ aspiration handpiece

CorCap cardiac support device

Cordis
    C. Bioptone sheath
    C. Checkmate system
    C-Hakim shunt
    C. Powerflex balloon catheter
    C. Predator PTCA balloon catheter

Cordis (*continued*)
  C. S.M.A.R.T. stent
  C. Trakstar PTCA balloon
    catheter

Core-Flex wire guides

Corin hip system

CorneaSparing LTK laser system

CoSeal resorbable synthetic
  sealant

cottonoid patty

Cournand cardiac device

Cragg
  C. Endopro stent system
  C. thrombolytic brush

Crutchfield skeletal traction
  tongs

CryoCare
  C. cardiac surgical system
  C. endometrial cryoablation
    system

Cryo/Cuff
  C. ankle dressing
  C. boot

CryoLife-O'Brien stentless
  porcine heart valve

cryophake

cryoprobe

cryostat

Cuda
  010L-100 laparoscope
  2510L-100 laparoscope

curet (*spelled also* curette)
  Abraham rectal c.
  Accurette endometrial
    suction c.
  adenoid c.
  Alvis foreign body eye c.
  Anderson c.
  Angell c.
  angled ring c.

curet (*continued*)
  antral c.
  aortic c.
  apicitis c.
  aspirating c.
  Austin oval c.
  Auto Suture c.
  B-12 dental c.
  Ballantine uterine c.
  Ballenger ethmoid c.
  banjo c.
  Bardic c.
  Barnhill adenoid c.
  Barnhill-Jones c.
  Barth mastoid c.
  bayonet c.
  Beaver c.
  Beckman adenoid c.
  Bellucci c.
  Berlin c.
  Billeau ear wax c.
  Billroth c.
  biopsy suction c.
  Blake uterine c.
  blunt-ring c.
  bone c.
  bowl c.
  box c.
  Bozeman c.
  Bromley uterine c.
  Bronson-Ray pituitary c.
  Brun bone c.
  Brun ear c.
  Brun mastoid c.
  Bruns bone c.
  Buck bone c.
  Buck ear c.
  Buck earring c.
  Buck mastoid c.
  Buck wax c.
  Buck-House c.
  Bumm placental c.
  Bumm uterine c.
  Bunge c.
  Bush intervertebral c.
  Carlens c.
  Carmack ear c.
  Carroll hook c.

curet (*continued*)
  Carter submucous c.
  cervical biopsy c.
  chalazion c.
  Charnley double-ended
    bone c.
  Clevedent-Lucas c.
  Cloward c.
  Cloward-Cone ring c.
  Clyman endometrial c.
  Coakley antral c.
  Coakley ethmoid c.
  Coakley nasal c.
  Coakley sinus c.
  Cobb bone c.
  Cobb spinal c.
  Collin uterine c.
  Concept c.
  Cone nasal c.
  Cone ring c.
  Cone suction biopsy c.
  Converse sweeper c.
  Corgill-Shapleigh ear c.
  corneal c.
  cup c.
  cupped c.
  curette forceps
  cylindrical uterine c.
  Daubenspeck bone c.
  Daviel chalazion c.
  Dawson-Yuhl c.
  Dawson-Yuhl-Cone c.
  DeLee c.
  Dench ear c.
  Dench uterine c.
  DePuy bone c.
  Derlacki ear c.
  dermal c.
  diagnostic c.
  disk c.
  disposable vacuum c.
  double-ended bone c.
  double-ended dental c.
  double-ended stapes c.
  double-lumen c.
  down-biting Epstein c.
  Duncan endometrial biopsy
    c.

curet (*continued*)
  Dunning c.
  ear c.
  embolectomy c.
  endaural c.
  endocervical biopsy c.
  endodontic c.
  endometrial c.
  endotracheal c.
  Epstein down-biting c.
  Epstein spinal fusion c.
  ethmoidal c.
  eye c.
  Farrior angulated c.
  Farrior ear c.
  Faulkner antral c.
  Faulkner double-end ring c.
  Faulkner ethmoidal c.
  Faulkner nasal c.
  fenestration c.
  Ferguson bone c.
  fine c.
  fine-angled c.
  Fink chalazion c.
  flat back c.
  foreign body c.
  fossa c.
  Fowler double-end c.
  Fox dermal c.
  Franklin-Silverman c.
  Freenseen rectal c.
  Freimuth ear c.
  Frenckner c.
  Frenckner-Stille c.
  frontal sinus c.
  Gam-Mer spinal fusion c.
  Garcia-Rock endometrial
    biopsy c.
  Genell biopsy c.
  Gifford corneal c.
  Gill-Welsh c.
  Gillquist suction c.
  Goldman c.
  Goldstein c.
  Goodhill double-end c.
  Govons pituitary c.
  Gracey c.
  Green corneal c.

curet (*continued*)

Greene endocervical c.
Greene placental c.
Greene uterine c.
Gross ear c.
Guilford-Wright c.
Gusberg cervical biopsy c.
Gusberg cervical cone c.
Gusberg endocervical
  biopsy c.
Halle bone c.
Halle ethmoidal c.
Halle sinus c.
Hannon endometrial c.
Hardy bayonet c.
Hardy hypophysial c.
Hardy modification of
  Bronson-Ray c.
Harrison-Shea c.
Hartmann adenoidal c.
Hatfield bone c.
Hayden tonsillar c.
Heaney endometrial biopsy
  c.
Heaney uterine c.
Heath chalazion c.
Hebra chalazion c.
Hebra corneal c.
Helix endocervical c.
Helix uterine biopsy c.
Heyner c.
Hibbs bone c.
Hibbs spinal c.
Hibbs-Spratt spinal fusion c.
Hofmeister endometrial
  biopsy c.
Holden uterine c.
Holtz endometrial c.
hook-type dermal c.
horizontal ring c.
Hough c.
House ear c.
House stapes c.
House tympanoplasty c.
House-Buck c.
House-Paparella stapes c.
House-Saunders middle ear
  c.

curet (*continued*)

House-Sheehy knife c.
Houtz endometrial c.
Howard spinal c.
Hunter uterine c.
hypophysial c.
Ingersoll adenoid c.
Innomed bone c.
intervertebral c.
irrigating uterine c.
Jacobson c.
Jansen bone c.
Jarit reverse adenoid c.
Jones adenoid c.
Jordan-Rosen c.
Juers ear c.
Kelly c.
Kelly-Gray uterine c.
Kerpel bone c.
Kevorkian endocervical c.
Kevorkian endometrial c.
Kevorkian-Younge
  endocervical biopsy c.
Kevorkian-Younge uterine
  c.
Kezerian c.
Kirkland c.
Kos c.
Kraff capsule polisher c.
Kuhn-Bolger angled c.
Kushner-Tandatnick
  endometrial biopsy c.
labyrinth c.
large bowel c.
large uterine c.
Laufe aspirating c.
Laufe-Novak diagnostic c.
Laufe-Novak gynecologic c.
Laufe-Randall gynecologic
  c.
Lempert bone c.
Lempert endaural c.
Lempert fine c.
long-handle c.
loop c.
Lounsbury placental c.
Lucas alveolar c.
Luer bone c.

curet (*continued*)

Luongo c.
Lynch c.
Magnum c.
Majewski nasal c.
Malis c.
Marino rotatable transsphenoidal horizontal-ring c.
Marino rotatable transsphenoidal vertical-ring c.
Marino transsphenoidal c.
Maroon lip c.
Martin dermal c.
Martini bone c.
mastoid c.
Mayfield spinal c.
McCain TMJ c.
McCaskey antral c.
McElroy c.
Meigs endometrial c.
Meigs uterine c.
meniscal c.
Meyerding saw-toothed c.
Meyhöffer bone c.
Meyhöffer chalazion c.
Mi-Mark disposable endocervical c.
microbone c.
Microsect c.
middle ear ring c.
Middleton adenoid c.
Milan uterine c.
Miles antral c.
Miller c.
Misdome-Frank c.
Mo-Mark c.
Moe bone c.
Molt c.
Moorfields c.
Mosher ethmoid c.
Moult c.
Mueller c.
Munchen endometrial biopsy c.
Myles antral c.
nasal c.

curet (*continued*)

Noland-Budd cervical c.
Nordent bone c.
Novak biopsy c.
Novak uterine c.
Novak-Schoeckaert endometrial c.
O'Connor double-edged c.
optical aspirating c.
Orban c.
orthopedic c.
oval-window c.
ovum c.
Paparella angled-ring c.
Paparella mastoid c.
Paparella stapes c.
Paparella-House c.
periapical c.
Piffard dermal c.
Piffard placental c.
Pipelle endometrial c.
Pipelle-deCornier endometrial c.
pituitary c.
placental c.
plastic c.
polyvinyl c.
Pratt antral c.
Pratt ethmoid c.
Pratt nasal c.
Récamier uterine c.
Rand bayonet ring c.
Randall endometrial biopsy c.
Randall uterine c.
Raney spinal fusion c.
Raney stirrup-loop c.
Ray pituitary c.
Read facial c.
Read oral c.
rectal c.
Reich c.
Reich-Nechtow cervical biopsy c.
Reiner c.
resectoscope c.
retrograde c.
reverse-angle skid c.

curet (*continued*)
        reverse-curve adenoid c.
        Rheinstaedter flushing c.
        Rheinstaedter uterine c.
        Rhoton blunt-ring c.
        Rhoton horizontal-ring c.
        Rhoton loop c.
        Rhoton pituitary c.
        Rhoton spoon c.
        Rhoton vertical ring c.
        Rica ear c.
        Rica lipoma c.
        Rica mastoid c.
        Rica uterine c.
        Richards bone c.
        Richards ethmoid c.
        Richards mastoid c.
        Ridpath ethmoid c.
        right-angle c.
        rigid c.
        ring bayonet Rand c.
        Rock endometrial suction
            c.
        Rosen knife c.
        Rosenmüller c.
        rotatable transsphenoidal
            horizontal ring c.
        rotatable transsphenoidal
            vertical ring c.
        ruptured disk c.
        salpingeal c.
        saw-toothed c.
        scarifying c.
        Schaefer ethmoid c.
        Schaefer mastoid c.
        Schede bone c.
        Schroeder uterine c.
        Schuletz antral c.
        Schuletz-Simmons
            ethmoidal c.
        Schwartz endocervical c.
        Scoville ruptured disk c.
        Semmes c.
        serrated c.
        Shambaugh adenoidal c.
        Shapleigh ear wax c.
        Sharman c.
        sharp dermal c.

curet (*continued*)
        sharp loop c.
        Shea c.
        Sheehy-House c.
        Simon bone c.
        Simon cup uterine c.
        Simon spinal c.
        Simpson antral c.
        Sims irrigating uterine c.
        sinus c.
        Skeele chalazion c.
        Skeele corneal c.
        Skeele eye c.
        skid c.
        Skillern sinus c.
        SMIC ear c.
        SMIC mastoid c.
        SMIC pituitary c.
        Smith-Petersen c.
        soft rubber c.
        sonic c.
        spinal fusion c.
        sponge ear c.
        spoon c.
        Sprague ear c.
        Spratt bone c.
        Spratt ear c.
        Spratt mastoid c.
        St. Clair-Thompson
            adenoidal c.
        stapes c.
        stirrup-loop c.
        Stiwer c.
        Storz resectoscope c.
        stout-neck c.
        straight ring c.
        Strully ruptured-disk c.
        Stubbs adenoidal c.
        submucous c.
        suction tip c.
        surgical c.
        Sweaper c.
        Synthes facial c.
        T-handled cup c.
        Tabb ear c.
        Tamsco c.
        Taylor c.
        Temens c.

curet (*continued*)
   Thomas uterine c.
   Thompson adenoid c.
   Thorpe c.
   tonsillar c.
   Townsend endocervical
      biopsy c.
   toxemia c.
   Toynbee c.
   transsphenoidal c.
   Uffenorde bone c.
   Ulbrich wart c.
   Ultra-Cut Cobb c.
   Unimar Pipelle c.
   up-angled c.
   uterine biopsy c.
   uterine irrigating c.
   uterine suction c.
   uterine vacuum aspirating
      c.
   Vabra suction c.
   Vacurette suction c.
   vacuum c.
   Vakutage c.
   vertical ring c.
   Visitec capsule polisher c.
   Vogel infant adenoid c.
   Volkmann bone c.
   Volkmann oval c.
   Voller c.
   Walker ring c.
   Walker ruptured-disk c.
   Wallich c.

curet (*continued*)
   Walsh dermal c.
   Walsh hook-type dermal c.
   Walton c.
   wax c.
   Weaver chalazion c.
   Weisman ear c.
   West-Beck spoon c.
   Whiting mastoid c.
   Whitney single-use plastic
      c.
   Williger bone c.
   Williger ear c.
   Wolf dermal c.
   Wright-Guilford c.
   Wullstein ring c.
   Yankauer ear c.
   Yankauer salpingeal c.
   Yasargil c.
   Younge endometrial c.
   Younge uterine c.
   Z-Sampler endometrial
      suction c.
   Zielke c.

curette (*variant of* curet)

C-wire Serter

cystitome (ophthalmology)

cystotome (urology)

Czaja-McCaffrey rigid stent
   introducer/endoscope

D

Dall-Miles cable grip system

defibrillator
  Angstrom II implantable
    cardioverter d.
  Angstrom MD implantable
    cardioverter d.
  Birtcher d.
  Cadence d.
  Cadet d.
  Cambridge d.
  Contour MD d.
  Contour Profile d.
  Contour V-145D d.
  Contour LTV-135D d.
  Endotak d.
  FirstSave automated
    external d.
  Forerunner d.
  Gem d.
  Guidant d.
  Heart Aid 80 d.
  Intec implantable d.
  IPCO-Partridge d.
  Jewel AF implantable d.
  Marquette Responder 1500
    multifuncitonal d.
  Medtronic GEM III
    implantable cardioverter d.
  Medtronic Jewel Plus Active
    Can d.
  Medtronic Micro Jewel d.
  ODAM d.
  Photon micro DR/VR
    implantable cardioverter
    d.
  Phylax 06 implantable
    cardioverter d.
  Porta Pulse 3 portable d.
  Prizm d.
  Ventak Mini III implantable
    d.
  Ventak Prizm implantable d.
  Zoll d.

Denver
  D. hydrocephalus shunt

Denver (*continued*)
  D. nasal splint
  D. PAK shunt
  D. pleuroperitoneal shunt
  D. reservoir
  D. valve
  D. valve shunt

Denver-Wells
  D.-W. atrial retractor
  D.-W. sternal retractor

DePuy
  D. AcroMed
  D. awl
  D. bolt
  D. Bremer AirFlo halo vest
    system
  D. cannulated reamer
  D. DOC Ventral Cervical
    Stabilization System
  D. fracture brace
  D. Lumbar I/V Cage
  D. ISOLA hook
  D. interference screw
  D. Kaneda smooth rod
    system
  D. Keystone graft
    instruments
  D. M-2 anterior plate system
  D. MOSS Miami hook
  D. PEAK anterior
    compression plate
  D. Profile system
  D. rocking leg splint
  D. rolled Colles splint
  D. Songer cable system
  D. SUMMIT rod
  D. TiMX Comprehensive
    Low Back System
  D. total hip system
  D. University plate system
  D. Vertigraft bone wedge
  D. VSP plate and screw
    system

Deschamps ligature carrier

Desilets-Hoffman introducer

Dialock access port

DiaPhine corneal trephination
device

Dilamezinsert urologic
instrument

dilator
Bakes common duct d.
Brown-McHardy pneumatic
d.
Garrett d.
Key-Med d.

Dingman otoplasty cartilage
abrader

dissection
Cavitron d.
Creed d.
Desmarres corneal d.
Dingman breast d.
Falcao suction d.
Kitner d.
Kuttner blunt d.
Neivert d.
Nezhat-Dorsey Trumpet
Valve hydrodissector
Pearce nucleus
hydrodissector
Rhoton d.
spud d.

dissector
dolphin nose d.
Maryland d.
SAPHfinder balloon d.
SAPHtrak balloon d.

Distaflo bypass graft

Diva laparoscopic morcellator

Dix-Hallpike position

Dobbhoff
D. biliary stent
D. gastrectomy feeding tube
D. PEG tube

Dohlman plug

DORC (Direct Optical Research
Company)
D. backflush instrument
D. handle
D. microforceps
D. vitreous shaver

Dornier
D. compact lithotripter
D. Epos Ultra lithotripter
D. HM-series lithotripter
D. scanner
D. Urotract cysto table

DoubleStent biliary
endoprosthesis

drain
Blair silicone d.
butterfly d.
Chaffin-Pratt d.
Clot Stop d.
Davol d.
J-Vac closed wound d.
Molteno implant d.
Nelaton rubber tube d.
Quad-Lumen d.
Relia-Vac d.
Shirley wound d.
Solcotrans closed vacuum
d.
Stryker d.
Thora-Drain III three-bottle
chest d.
Thora-Klex chest d.

drapes
Abandia d.

dressing
AcryDerm d.
AcryDerm border island d.
Acticoat silver-based burn
d.
Acu-Derm IV/TPN d.
Acu-Derm wound d.
AlgiDERM alginate wound d.
AlgiSite alginate wound d.
Algosteril alginate wound d.
Alldress d.

dressing (*continued*)
    Allevyn d.
    Aquacel Hydrofiber d.
    Aquasorb transparent
      hydrogel d.
    ArtAssist d.
    Bioclusive transparent d.
    Biopatch foam wound d.
    BlisterFilm transparent d.
    BreakAway absorptive
      wound d.
    CarraFilm transparent d.
    CarraSmart foam d.
    Carra Sorb H d.
    Carra Sorb M. d.
    Carrasyn Hydrogel d.
    Catrix d.
    CicaCare topical gel sheet
      d.
    CircPlus compression d.
    Circulon d.
    ClearSite borderless d.
    ClearSite Hydro Gauze d.
    Coban d.
    CollaCote collagen wound
      d.
    CollaPlug d.
    CombiDerm d.
    Comfeel Ulcus occlusive d.
    Composite Cultured Skin
    Conformant d.
    Covaderm composite
      wound d.
    Coverlet adhesive d.
    Cover-Roll d.
    Cryo/Cuff ankle d.
    Curaderm d.
    Curafil d.
    Curafoam d.
    Curagel Hydrogel d.
    Curasorb calcium alginate
      d.
    Cutinova Cavity d.
    Cutinova Hydro d.
    Dermacea alginate wound
      d.
    Dermagran hydrophilic
      wound d.

dressing (*continued*)
    DermaMend foam wound d.
    DermaMend hydrogel d.
    DermaNet contact-layer
      wound d.
    DermAssist hydrocolloid d.
    Dermatell hydrocolloid d.
    DiabGel hydrogel d.
    DuoDerm compression d.
    DynaFlex compression d.
    Elastikon elastic tape d.
    Elasto-Gel hydrogel d.
    Elta Dermal hydrogel d.
    EpiFilm otologic lamina d.
    Epi-lock polyurethane foam
      wound d.
    ExuDerm hydrocolloid d.
    Exu-Dry absorptive d.
    Firbracol collagen-alginate d.
    Flexzan foam wound d.
    FortaDerm d.
    Fuller shield d.
    FyBron alginate d.
    Gentell alginate wound d.
    Gentell foam wound d.
    GraftCyte d.
    hyCure collagen hemostatic
      wound d.
    Hydrocol d.
    Hypergel d.
    Iamin Gel wound d.
    Inerpan d.
    Intelligent d.
    IntraSite gel d.
    Iodoflex absorptive d.
    Iodosorb absorptive d.
    Kalginate alginate wound d.
    Kaltostat wound d.
    Liquiderm d.
    Lyofoam d.
    Maxorb alginate wound d.
    Mefilm d.
    Melgisorb calcium alginate d.
    Mepiform d.
    Mepilex d.
    Mepitel d.
    Merogel nasal d. and sinus
      stent

dressing (*continued*)
>Mitraflex d.
Normigel hydrogel d.
N-Terface contact-layer
>wound d.
Oasis wound d.
O'Donoghue d.
OpSite Flexigrid transparent
>adhesive film d.
OsmoCyte pillow d.
Oxiplex
PanoGauze hydrogel-
>impregnated gauze d.
PanoPlex hydrogel d.
Pillo Pro d.
PolyMem wound care d.
Polyskin II d.
Primapore absorptive
>wound d.
ProClude transparent
>adhesive film d.
ProCyte transparent
>adhesive film d.
Profore four-layer bandage
PuraPly wound d.
RepliCare hydrocolloid d.
Repliderm d.
Reston foam wound d.
Restore alginate wound d.
Saf-Gel hydrogel d.
SeaSorb alginate wound d.
SignaDRESS hydrocolloid d.
Silon wound d.
Silverlon wound packing
>strips
SIS wound d.
SiteGuard MVP transparent
>adhesive film d.
SkinTegrity hydrogel d.
SofSorb absorptive d.
SoftCloth absorptive d
Sorbsan topical wound d.
Spyrogel hydrogel wound d.
Stratasorb composite
>wound d.

dressing (*continued*)
>SureSite transparent
>adhesive film d.
Synthaderm d.
Tegaderm transparent d.
Tegagel hydrogel d.
Tegagen alginate wound d.
Tegapore contact-layer
>wound d.
THINSite d.
THINSite with Bio/film
>hydrogel topical wound d.
Tielle absorptive d.
Transeal transparent
>adhesive film d.
Unna-Flex compression d.
Unna-Pak compression d.
Ultec hydrocolloid d.
Ultrafera wound d.
Veingard d.
Velpeau d.
Viasorb d.
Vigilon d.
Woun'Dres hydrogel d.
Xeroform d.
Zipzoc stocking
>compression d.

drill
>Fisch d.
Gray bone d.

Dua stent

Duett vascular sealing device

Duette
>D. basket
D. catheter
D. double lumen ERCP
>instrument
D. probe

Du Pen catheter

Durasul
>D. hip prosthesis
D. knee prosthesis

Eagle straight-ahead
  arthroscope

Earle
    E. hemorrhoidal clamp
    E. rectal probe

Easi-Lav gastric lavage system

Easy Rider microcatheter

Eccentric Y retractor

EchoSeed brachytherapy
  seed/implant

Eder
    E.-Puestow esophageal
      dilator
    E.-Puestow guidewire

Edna
    E. towel clamp
    E. towel forceps

Edslab
    E. cholangiography catheter
    E. jaw spring clip

Edwards Prima Plus valve

Eggers
    E. bone plate
    E. screw

Eisenstein
    E. clamp
    E. hysterectomy forceps

electrode
    Aspen laparoscopic e.
    Bard-Hamm fulgurating e.
    BICAP monopolar e.
    CapSure e.
    Clarion HiFocus e.
    Coaguloop resection e.
    coude fulgurating e.
    Eppendorf needle e.
    EVAP roller e.
    Hymes-Timberlake e.
    Iglesias e.
    iontophoresis e.

electrode (*continued*)
    LLETZ/LEEP loop e.
    Quinton Quik-Prep e.
    roller-bar e.
    roller-barrel e.
    round-loop e.
    round-wire e.
    Storz cystoscopic e.
    Storz resectoscope e.
    Teq-Trode e.
    Timberlake e.
    Turner cystoscopic
      fulgurating e.
    Uroloop e.
    Valleylab ball e.
    Valleylab loop e.
    VaporTome resection e.
    VaporTrode roller e.

elevator
    Adson periosteal e.
    Allerdyce e.
    Aufranc periosteal e.
    Aufricht e.
    Bellucci e.
    Bristow periosteal e.
    Cinelli periosteal e.
    Cloward osteophyte e.
    Cloward periosteal e.
    Cottle e.
    Cottle-McKenty e.
    Cronin palate e.
    Davidson-Mathieu-
      Alexander periosteal e.
    Dingman periosteal e.
    Doyen costal e.
    Ellik e.
    Endotrac e.
    Farabeuf periosteal e.
    Freer double-end e.
    Goldman septal e.
    Hajek-Ballenger septal e.
    Hough hoe e.
    Hulka-Kenwick uterine e.
    Jarit periosteal e.
    Joseph-Killian septal e.

elevator (*continued*)
    Kinsella periosteal e.
    Luongo septal e.
    MacKenty septal e.
    Norrbacka bone e.
    Paparella duckbill e.
    Pennington septal e.
    Pollock zygoma e.
    Rhoton e.
    Richards-Cobb spinal e.
    Sokolec e.
    Somer uterine e.
    Soonawalla uterine e.
    Stille-Langenbeck e.
    Urquhart periosteal e.
    zygoma e.

Eliminator
    E. ArthroWand
    E. biliary stent
    E. pancreatic stent
    E. stone extraction basket

Ellik
    E. bladder evacuator
    E. kidney stone basket
    E. loop stone dislodger
    E. resectoscope

Elmor tissue morcellator

embarc bone repair material

Embryon
    E. GIFT transfer catheter
    E. HSG catheter

EnAbl thermal ablation system

Ender
    E. fixation
    E. nail
    E. rod

Endius spinal endoscope

Endo-AID suction irrigation

Endo-Assist
    E.-A. endoscopic forceps
    E.-A. endoscopic knot
        pusher

Endo-Assist
    E.-A. endoscopic ligature
        carrier
    E.-A. endoscopic needle
        holder
    E.-A. retractable blade
    E.-A. retractable scalpel
    E.-A. sponge aspirator

Endobag specimen bag

EndoCinch suturing system

EndoCatch

Endo Clip applier

Endocut cautery device

Endodissect reticulating
    dissecting instrument

EndoFix absorbable
    interference screw

Endo Grasp device

Endo-Hernia stapler

Endoloop disposable chromic
    ligature suture instrument

EndoMate Grab Bag specimen
    retrieval bag

Endopath
    E. disposable surgical trocar
    E. EMS hernia stapler
    E. ES reusable endoscopic
        stapler
    E. ETS-FLEX endoscopic
        articulating linear cutter
    E. EZ45 endoscopic linear
        cutter
    E. EZ45 No Knife
        endoscopic linear cutter
    E. EZ-RF linear cutter and
        coagulation device
    E. laparoscopic trocar
    E. Optiview optical surgical
        obturator
    E. Stealth stapler
    E. TriStar trocar
    E. Ultra Veress needle

Endopouch Pro specimen-
  retrieval bag

Endosac seamless specimen
  collection pouch

endoscope
  Agee e.
  AO indirect
    ophthalmoscope
  Baggish hysteroscope
  Benjamin pediatric
    laryngoscope
  CF-200Z Olympus
    colonoscope
  Digiscope
  falloposcope
  Flexiblade laryngoscope
  Futura resectoscope sheath
  Gautier ureteroscope
  InjecTx cystoscope
  Kantor-Berci video
    laryngoscope
  Killian-Lynch laryngoscope
  Kuda e.
  Lewy suspension
    laryngoscope
  Lindholm operating
    laryngoscope
  MicroLap e.
  MiniSite laparoscope
  Morganstern continuous-
    flow operating cystoscope
  Navigator flexible
    endoscope
  oblique-viewing e.
  Ossoff-Karlen laryngoscope
  Pentax side-viewing e.
  Pixie minilaparoscope
  Rockey e.
  Sensatec e.
  Sine-U-View nasal
    endoscope
  Sonde enteroscope
  Surgenomic e.
  Toshiba video e.
  variable stiffness e.
  VideoHydro laparoscope
  Visicath e.

endoscope (*continued*)
  Welch Allyn video e.
  Zeiss Endolive e.

EndoShears

Endo Stitch suturing device

Endotak
  E. Endurance EZ lead
  E. Endurance Rx lead
  E. Reliance defibrillator
    lead

Endotrac
  E. cannula
  E. elevator
  E. obturator
  E. probe
  E. rasp
  E. retractor

EpiFilm

Epistat double balloon

Equinox occlusion balloon
  system

eraser
  e. cautery
  hemostatic e.
  Mentor Curved e.
  Mentor Wet-Field e.
  Tano e.

Erich
  E. arch malleable bar
  E. laryngeal biopsy forceps
  E. maxillary splint
  E. nasal splint
  E. swivel

Escort balloon stone extractor

Evac device

EVAP roller electrode

Evershears
  E. bipolar curved scissors
  E. bipolar laparoscopic
    forceps
  E. bipolar laparoscopic
    scissors

Evershears (*continued*)
    E. surgical instrument
        device

Eves-Neivert tonsillar snare

Ewald
    E. gastroscope
    E. tissue forceps
    E. tube

Exeter intramedullary bone
    plug

expander
    AccuSpan tissue e.
    Becker tissue e.
    Integra tissue e.
    McGhan tissue e.

expander (*continued*)
    Mentor tissue e.
    Meshgraft skin e.
    Radovan tissue e.
    saline-filled e.
    subperiosteal tissue e.
    T-Span tissue e.

Extra View balloon

eXtract specimen bag

ExtreSafe
    E. butterfly
    E. catheter
    E. lancet
    E. needle
    E. syringe

Falope ring

falloposcope

FASTak suture anchor system

fat towel

FemoStop femoral artery
compression device

Filcard temporary removable
vena cava filter

filter
bird's nest f.
Rubicon embolic f.
TrapEase f.

Filshie femoral sterilization clip

Fine-Thornton scleral fixation
ring

Fisch drill

FlashPoint image-guided
surgical instruments

Fletcher-Suit applicator

Fletcher-Suit-Delclos colpostat

Flexiflo
F. Lap G laparoscopic
gastrostomy kit
F. Lap J laparoscopic
jejunostomy kit
F. Stomate low-profile
gastrostomy tube

Flieringa sclera ring

Flo-Restor backbleeding device

FloSeal matrix hemostatic
sealant

Florida pouch

FlowGun suction/irrigation

Fluoropassiv thin-wall carotid
patch

FocalSeal liquid sealant

forceps
Abbott-Mayfield f.
Abernaz strut f.
abscess f.
Absolok f.
ACMI Martin endoscopic f.
Acufex curved basket f.
Acufex rotary basket f.
Acufex straight basket f.
AcuTouch tissue f.
Adair tissue
Adair tissue-holding f.
Adair uterine f.
Adair-Allis tissue f.
adenoid
Adler bone f.
Adler punch f.
Adler-Kreutz f.
adnexal f.
Adson arterial f.
Adson bayonet dressing f.
Adson bipolar f.
Adson brain f.
Adson clip-applying f.
Adson dressing f.
Adson hemostatic f.
Adson hypophyseal f.
Adson microbipolar f.
Adson microdressing f.
Adson microtissue f.
Adson monopolar f.
Adson scalp clip-applying f.
Adson thumb f.
Adson tissue f.
Adson tooth f.
Adson-Biemer f.
Adson-Brown f.
Adson-Brown tissue f.
Adson-Callison tissue f.
Adson-Mixter neurosurgical
f.
Adson-Vital tissue f.
advancement f.
Aesculap f.
Akins valve re-do f.
Alabama University f.

forceps (*continued*)

    Alderkreutz tissue f.
    Alexander dressing f.
    Alexander-Farabeuf f.
    Allen intestinal f.
    Allen uterine f.
    Allen-Barkan f.
    Allen-Braley f.
    alligator crimper f.
    alligator cup f.
    alligator ear f.
    alligator nasal f.
    Allis delicate tissue f.
    Allis intestinal f.
    Allis Micro-Line pediatric f.
    Allis thoracic f.
    Allis-Abramson breast
      biopsy f.
    Allis-Adair intestinal f.
    Allis-Adair tissue f.
    Allis-Coakley tonsil-seizing
      f.
    Allis-Coakley tonsillar f.
    Allis-Duval f.
    Allis-Ochsner tissue f.
    Allis-Ochsner tonsillar f.
    Allis-Willauer tissue f.
    Almeida f.
    Alvis fixation f.
    Ambrose eye f.
    Ambrose suture f.
    Amdur lid f.
    Amenabar capsular f.
    American Catheter Corp.
      biopsy f.
    AMO phacoemulsification
      lens-folder f.
    anastomosis f.
    Andrews tonsil-seizing f.
    Andrews tonsillar f.
    Andrews-Hartmann f.
    aneurysm f.
    Angell-James
      hypophysectomy f.
    Angell-James punch f.
    angiotribe f.
    angled capsular f.
    angled stone f.

forceps (*continued*)

    Anis capsulotomy f.
    Anis corneal f.
    Anis corneoscleral f.
    Anis intraocular lens f.
    Anis microsurgical tying f.
    Anis straight corneal f.
    Anis tying f.
    anterior capsule f.
    anterior segment f.
    Anthony-Fisher f.
    antral f.
    aortic aneurysm f.
    aortic occlusion f.
    Apfelbaum bipolar f.
    Apple Medical bipolar f.
    applicator f.
    approximation f.
    Archer splinter f.
    Arrow articulation paper f.
    Arrowsmith fixation f.
    Arrowsmith-Clerf pin-
      closing f.
    Arroyo f.
    Arruga curved capsular f.
    Arruga-Gill f.
    Arruga-McCool capsular f.
    arterial f.
    Arthro Force basket cutting
      f.
    Arthur splinter f.
    articulating paper f.
    Artilk f.
    Asch septal f.
    Asch septum-straightening
      f.
    Ash dental f.
    Ash septum-straightening f.
    Ashby fluoroscopic foreign
      body f.
    ASSI bipolar coagulating f.
    Athens f.
    atraumatic tissue f.
    atraumatic visceral f.
    aural f.
    auricular appendage f.
    Austin f.
    Auto Suture f.

forceps (*continued*)
  Autraugrip tissue f.
  Auvard-Zweifel f.
  axis-traction f.
  Ayers chalazion f.
  Azar intraocular f.
  Azar lens f.
  Azar tying f.
  Azar utility f.
  B-H f.
  B-P transfer f.
  Babcock intestinal f.
  Babcock lung-grasping f.
  Babcock thoracic tissue f.
  Babcock thoracic tissue-
    holding f.
  Babcock-Beasley f.
  Babcock-Vital atraumatic f.
  Babcock-Vital intestinal f.
  Babcock-Vital tissue f.
  baby Adson f.
  baby Allis f.
  baby Crile f.
  baby dressing f.
  baby hemostatic f.
  baby intestinal tissue f.
  baby Lane bone-holding f.
  baby Mikulicz f.
  baby Mixter f.
  baby mosquito f.
  baby Overholt f.
  backbiting f.
  Backhaus f.
  Backhaus-Roeder f.
  Bacon cranial f.
  Baer bone-cutting f.
  Bahnson-Brown f.
  Bailey aortic valve-cutting f.
  Bailey chalazion f.
  Bailey-Williamson
    obstetrical f.
  Bainbridge hemostatic f.
  Bainbridge intestinal f.
  Bainbridge resection f.
  Bainbridge thyroid f.
  Baird chalazion f.
  Baker tissue f.
  Ball f.

forceps (*continued*)
  Ballantine hysterectomy f.
  Ballantine-Peterson
    hysterectomy f.
  Ballen-Alexander f.
  Ballenger hysterectomy f.
  Ballenger sponge f.
  Ballenger tonsillar f.
  Ballenger-Foerster f.
  Bane rongeur f.
  Bangerter muscle f.
  Banner f.
  Bansal LASIK f.
  Bard f.
  Bard-Parker f.
  Bardeleben bone-holding f.
  Barkan iris f.
  Barlow f.
  Barnes-Crile hemostatic f.
  Barnes-Hill f.
  Barnes-Simpson obstetrical
    f.
  Baron f.
  Barracuda flexible
    cystoscopic hot biopsy f.
  Barraquer ciliary f.
  Barraquer conjunctival f.
  Barraquer corneal f.
  Barraquer fixation f.
  Barraquer hemostatic
    mosquito f.
  Barraquer-Katzin f.
  Barraquer-Troutman
    corneal f.
  Barraquer-von Mandach
    capsule f.
  Barraquer-von Mandach
    clot f.
  Barraya tissue f.
  Barrett intestinal f.
  Barrett lens f.
  Barrett placental f.
  Barrett tenacular f.
  Barrett-Allen placental f.
  Barrett-Allen uterine f.
  Barrett-Murphy intestinal f.
  Barrie-Jones angled
    crocodile f.

forceps (*continued*)

Barron alligator f.
Barsky f.
Barton obstetrical f.
basket f.
basket-cutting f.
basket-punch f.
basket-type crushing f.
Bauer dissecting f.
Bauer sponge f.
Baum-Hecht tarsorrhaphy f.
Baumberger f.
Baumgartner f.
Bausch articulation paper f.
bayonet bipolar f.
bayonet monopolar f.
bayonet root tip f.
BB shot f.
Bead ethmoidal f.
beaked cowhorn f.
bean f.
Beardsley f.
bearing-seating f.
Beasley-Babcock tissue f.
Beaupre ciliary f.
Beaupre epilation f.
Bechert lens-holding f.
Bechert-McPherson tying f.
Beck f.
Beebe hemostatic f.
Beebe wire-cutting f.
Beer ciliary f.
Behen ear f.
Behrend cystic duct f.
Bellucci ear f.
Benaron scalp-rotating f.
Bengolea arterial f.
Bennell f.
Bennett ciliary f.
Bennett epilation f.
Berens capsular f.
Berens corneal transplant f.
Berens muscle recession f.
Berens ptosis f.
Berens recession f.
Berens suturing f.
Berger biopsy f.
Bergeron pillar f.

forceps (*continued*)

Bergh ciliary f.
Berghmann-Foerster
   sponge f.
Bergman tissue f.
Berke ciliary f.
Berke ptosis f.
Berkeley Bioengineering
   ptosis f.
Bernard uterine f.
Berne nasal f.
Bernhard towel f.
Berry uterine-elevating f.
Best common duct
   stone f.
Best gallstone f.
Bettman-Noyes fixation f.
Bevan gallbladder f.
Bevan hemostatic f.
Beyer f.
Bi-tec f.
BiCoag bipolar
   laparoscopic f.
Bierer ovum f.
Bigelow f.
Bill traction handle f.
Billroth uterine tumor f.
Binkhorst lens f.
binocular fixation f.
biopsy punch f.
biopsy specimen f.
bipolar bayonet f.
bipolar coagulating f.
bipolar coaptation f.
bipolar cutting f.
bipolar electrocautery f.
bipolar eye f.
bipolar irrigating f.
bipolar laparoscopic f.
bipolar long-shaft f.
bipolar suction f.
bipolar transsphenoidal f.
Bircher-Ganske meniscal
   cartilage f.
Bireks dissecting f.
Birkett hemostatic f.
Birks Mark II Colibri f.
Birks Mark II grooved f.

forceps (*continued*)

Birks Mark II microneedle-
holder f.
Birks Mark II needle-holder
f.
Birks Mark II straight f.
Birks Mark II suture-tying f.
Birks Mark II toothed f.
Birtcher endoscopic f.
Bishop tissue f.
Bishop-Harman dressing f.
Bishop-Harman foreign
body f.
Bishop-Harman iris f.
Bishop-Harman tissue f.
bite biopsy f.
biting f.
Björk diathermy f.
Björk-Stille diathermy f.
bladder specimen f.
Blade-Wilde ear f.
Blake dressing f.
Blake ear f.
Blake embolus f.
Blake gallstone f.
Blakesley ethmoid f.
Blakesley septal bone f.
Blakesley septal
compression f.
Blakesley-Weil upturned
ethmoid f.
Blakesley-Wilde ear f.
Blakesley-Wilde nasal f.
Blalock f.
Blalock-Kleinert f.
Blanchard hemorrhoidal f.
Bland cervical traction f.
Bland vulsellum f.
Blaydes angled lens f.
Blaydes corneal f.
Blaydes lens-holding f.
blepharochalasis f.
Block-Potts intestinal f.
Blohmka tonsillar f.
Bloodwell tissue f.
Bloodwell vascular f.
Bloodwell-Brown f.
Bloomberg lens f.

forceps (*continued*)

Blum f.
Blumenthal uterine
dressing f.
blunt f.
Boer craniotomy f.
Boerma obstetrical f.
Boettcher arterial f.
Boettcher pulmonary artery
f.
Boettcher tonsillar artery f.
Boettcher-Schnidt f.
Boies cutting f.
Bolton f.
Bonaccolto cup jaws f.
Bonaccolto fragment f.
Bonaccolto jeweler's f.
Bonaccolto magnet tip f.
Bonaccolto utility f.
Bond placental f.
bone punch f.
bone-biting f.
bone-cutting double-action
f.
bone-holding f.
bone-reduction f.
bone-splitting f.
Bonn European suturing f.
Bonn iris f.
Bonn peripheral iridectomy
f.
Bonn suturing f.
Bonney tissue f.
Bores corneal fixation f.
Bores U-shaped f.
Boruchoff f.
Boston Lying-In cervical f.
Botvin iris f.
Botvin vulsellum f.
Bouchayer grasping f.
Bovie coagulating f.
Bovino scleral-spreading f.
bowel f.
Bowen suction loose body
f.
box-joint f.
Boys-Allis tissue f.
Bozeman LR dressing f.

forceps (*continued*)

Bozeman LR packing f.
Bozeman LR uterine-
   dressing f.
Bozeman uterine f.
Bozeman uterine-dressing f.
Bozeman uterine-packing f.
Bozeman-Douglas dressing
   f.
Braasch bladder specimen
   f.
Bracken fixation f.
Bracken iris f.
Bracken scleral fixation f.
Bracken-Forkas corneal f.
Bradford thyroid f.
brain clip f.
brain dressing f.
brain spatula f.
brain tissue f.
brain tumor f.
Braithwaite f.
Brand passing f.
Brand shunt-introducing f.
Brand tendon-holding f.
Brand tendon-passing f.
Braun f.
Brenner f.
Bridge deep-surgery f.
Bridge hemostatic f.
Bridge intestinal f.
Brigham 1×2 teeth f.
Brigham brain tumor f.
Brigham dressing f.
Brigham thumb tissue f.
Brock biopsy f.
bronchial biopsy f.
bronchial-grasping f.
bronchoscopic biopsy f.
bronchus-grasping f.
Bronson-Magnion f.
Brophy dressing f.
Brophy tissue f.
Brown side-grasping f.
Brown thoracic f.
Brown tissue f.
Brown-Adson side-grasping
   f.

forceps (*continued*)

Brown-Bahnson bayonet f.
Brown-Buerger f.
Brown-Cushing f.
Brown-Swan f.
Broyles optical f.
Bruening cutting-tip f.
Bruening ethmoid
   exenteration f.
Bruening nasal-cutting
   septal f.
Bruening septal f.
Bruening-Citelli f.
Brunner intestinal f.
Brunner sigmoid
   anastomosis f.
Brunner tissue f.
Brunschwig arterial f.
Brunschwig visceral f.
Bryant nasal f.
Buck foreign body f.
Buerger-McCarthy bladder
   f.
Buie biopsy f.
Buie rectal f.
Buie specimen f.
bulldog clamp-applying f.
bullet f.
Bumpus specimen f.
Bunim urethral f.
Bunker modification of
   Jackson laryngeal f.
Buratto flap f.
Buratto LASIK f.
Buratto ophthalmic f.
Burch biopsy f.
Burford coarctation f.
Burnham biopsy f.
Burns bone f.
Butler bayonet f.
Bycep biopsy f.
C. L. Jackson head-holding
   f.
C. L. Jackson pin-bending
   costophrenic f.
Cairns dissection f.
Cairns hemostatic f.
Cairns-Dandy hemostasis f.

forceps (*continued*)
- Calibri f.
- Callahan scleral fixation f.
- Callison-Adson tissue f.
- Cameron-Miller type monopolar f.
- Campbell ligature-carrier f.
- Campbell ureteral f.
- Cane bone-holding f.
- cannulated bronchoscopic f.
- capsular f.
- capsule-grasping f.
- capsulorhexis f.
- capsulotomy f.
- caput f.
- Carb-Bite tissue f.
- carbide-jaw f.
- Cardio-Grip iliac f.
- Cardio-Grip tissue f.
- cardiovascular tissue f.
- Cardona corneal prosthesis f.
- Cardona threading lens f.
- Carlens f.
- Carmalt arterial f.
- Carmalt hemostatic f.
- Carmalt hysterectomy f.
- Carmalt splinter f.
- Carmalt thoracic f.
- Carmody thumb tissue f.
- Carmody-Brophy f.
- carotid artery f.
- Carrel hemostatic f.
- Carrel mosquito f.
- Carroll bone-holding f.
- Carroll dressing f.
- Carroll tendon-passing f.
- Carroll tendon-pulling f.
- Carroll tissue f.
- Carroll-Adson dural f.
- cartilage f.
- cartilage-holding f.
- Cartman lens insertion f.
- caruncle f.
- Caspar alligator f.
- Cassidy-Brophy dressing f.
- Castaneda vascular f.

forceps (*continued*)
- Castaneda-Mixter f.
- Castroviejo capsular f.
- Castroviejo capsule f.
- Castroviejo clip-applying f.
- Castroviejo cornea-holding f.
- Castroviejo corneoscleral f.
- Castroviejo cross-action capsular f.
- Castroviejo eye suture f.
- Castroviejo fixation f.
- Castroviejo lid f.
- Castroviejo scleral fold f.
- Castroviejo suture f.
- Castroviejo suturing f.
- Castroviejo transplant f.
- Castroviejo transplant-grafting f.
- Castroviejo tying f.
- Castroviejo wide grip handle f.
- Castroviejo-Arruga capsular f.
- Castroviejo-Colibri corneal f.
- Castroviejo-Furness cornea-holding f.
- Castroviejo-Simpson f.
- Catalano capsular f.
- Catalano corneoscleral f.
- Catalano tying f.
- catheter-introducing f.
- Cavanaugh-Wells tonsillar f.
- center-action f.
- cephalic blade f.
- cervical biopsy f.
- cervical grasping f.
- cervical hemostatic f.
- cervical punch f.
- cervical traction f.
- cesarean f.
- chalazion f.
- Chamberlen obstetrical f.
- Championnière f.
- Chandler iris f.
- Chandler spinal-perforating f.

forceps (*continued*)

Chang bone-cutting f.
Chaput tissue f.
Charnley suture f.
Charnley wire-holding f.
Charnley-Riches arterial f.
Cheatle sterilizing f.
Cheron uterine dressing f.
Cherry f.
Cherry-Adson f.
Cherry-Kerrison f.
Chester sponge f.
Chevalier Jackson
    bronchoesophagoscopy f.
chicken-bill rongeur f.
Child clip-applying f.
Child intestinal f.
Child-Phillips f.
Children's Hospital
    dressing f.
Children's Hospital
    intestinal f.
Chimani pharyngeal f.
Choyce intraocular lens f.
Choyce lens-inserting f.
Christopher-Stille f.
Chubb tonsillar f.
Cicherelli f.
Cilco lens f.
cilia suture f.
Circon Tripolar f.
circular cup bronchoscopic
    biopsy f.
Citelli punch f.
Citelli-Bruening ear f.
Civiale f.
clamp f.
Clark capsule fragment f.
Clark ligator scissor f.
Clark-Guyton f.
Clark-Verhoeff
    capsular f.
claw f.
Clayman corneal f.
Clayman lens f.
Clayman lens-holding f.
Clayman lens-inserting f.
Clayman suturing f.

forceps (*continued*)

Clayman-Kelman
    intraocular lens f.
Clayman-McPherson tying f.
cleft palate f.
Clemetson uterine f.
Clerf f.
Clevedent f.
Cleveland bone-cutting f.
clip f.
clip-applying aneurysm f.
clip-bending f.
clip-cutting f.
clip-introducing f.
clip-removing f.
closed iris f.
closer f.
closing f.
clot f.
coagulating f.
coagulation f.
Coakley tonsillar f.
Coakley-Allis tonsillar f.
coaptation bipolar f.
coarctation f.
coated biopsy f.
Cobaugh eye f.
Codman fallopian tube f.
Codman ovary f.
Cohen corneal f.
Cohen nasal-dressing f.
cold biopsy f.
cold cup biopsy f.
Coleman-Taylor IOL f.
Colibri corneal f.
Colibri eye f.
Colibri-Pierse f.
Colibri-Storz corneal f.
College f.
Coller arterial f.
Coller hemostatic f.
Colley tissue f.
Colley traction f.
Collier hemostatic f.
Collier-Crile hemostatic f.
Collier-DeBakey hemostatic
    f.
Collin dressing f.

forceps (*continued*)

Collin intestinal f.
Collin lung-grasping f.
Collin mucous f.
Collin ovarian f.
Collin tissue f.
Collin tongue f.
Collin tongue-seizing f.
Collin uterine-elevating f.
Collin-Duval intestinal f.
Collin-Duval-Crile intestinal f.
Collin-Pozzi uterine f.
Collis-Maumenee corneal f.
Coloviras-Rumel thoracic f.
Colver tonsil-seizing f.
Colver tonsillar pillar-grasping f.
Colver-Coakley tonsillar f.
common duct stone f.
common duct-holding f.
common McPherson f.
compression f.
Cone wire-twisting f.
conjunctival fixation f.
connector f.
contact compressive f.
continuous clip f.
Cook flexible biopsy f.
Cooley anastomosis f.
Cooley aortic f.
Cooley arterial occlusion f.
Cooley auricular appendage f.
Cooley cardiovascular f.
Cooley coarctation f.
Cooley curved f.
Cooley double-angled jaw f.
Cooley graft f.
Cooley iliac f.
Cooley neonatal vascular f.
Cooley patent ductus f.
Cooley pediatric aortic f.
Cooley peripheral vascular f.
Cooley tangential pediatric f.
Cooley tissue f.

forceps (*continued*)

Cooley vascular tissue f.
Cooley-Baumgarten aortic f.
Cooley-Derra anastomosis f.
Cope lung f.
Coppridge grasping f.
Coppridge urethral f.
Corbett bone-cutting f.
Cordes esophagoscopy f.
Cordes-New laryngeal punch f.
Corey ovum f.
Corey placental f.
Corgill-Hartmann f.
cornea-holding f.
cornea-suturing f.
corneal fixation f.
corneal prosthesis f.
corneal splinter f.
corneal transplant f.
corneal utility f.
corneoscleral suturing f.
Cornet f.
coronary artery f.
Corson myoma f.
Corwin tonsillar f.
Cottle biting f.
Cottle insertion f.
Cottle lower lateral f.
Cottle tissue f.
Cottle-Arruga cartilage f.
Cottle-Jansen f.
Cottle-Kazanjian bone-cutting f.
Cottle-Kazanjian nasal f.
Cottle-Walsham septum-straightening f.
cowhorn tooth-extracting f.
Cozean angled lens f.
Cozean bipolar f.
Cozean implantation f.
Cozean-McPherson angled lens f.
Cozean-McPherson tying f.
Crafoord arterial f.
Crafoord bronchial f.
Crafoord coarctation f.
Crafoord pulmonary f.

forceps (*continued*)

    Crafoord-Sellors hemostatic f.
    Craig nasal-cutting f.
    Craig septal f.
    Craig septum bone-cutting f.
    Craig tonsil-seizing f.
    cranial f.
    cranium clip-applying f.
    Crawford fascial f.
    Crawford-Knighton f.
    Creevy biopsy f.
    Crenshaw caruncle f.
    Crile arterial f.
    Crile gall duct f.
    Crile hemostatic f.
    Crile Micro-Line arterial f.
    Crile-Barnes hemostatic f.
    Crile-Duval lung-grasping f.
    Crile-Rankin f.
    crimper f.
    crimping f.
    Crockard ligament grasping f.
    Crockard odontoid peg-grasping f.
    crocodile biopsy f.
    cross-action capsular f.
    Crossen puncturing tenaculum f.
    crural nipper f.
    Cryer Universal f.
    CSF shunt-introducing f.
    Cukier nasal f.
    Culler eye f.
    Culler fixation f.
    Cullom septal f.
    cup biopsy f.
    cup-biting f.
    cup-shaped curette f.
    cup-shaped inner ear f.
    cup-shaped middle ear f.
    cupped f.
    curette f.
    Curtis tissue f.
    curved dissecting f.
    curved iris f.

forceps (*continued*)

    curved knot-tying f.
    curved Maryland f.
    curved microbipolar f.
    curved micromonopolar f.
    curved tying f.
    curved-tip jeweler's bipolar f.
    Cushing bayonet f.
    Cushing bipolar neurosurgical f.
    Cushing brain f.
    Cushing cranial rongeur f.
    Cushing decompression f.
    Cushing dressing f.
    Cushing monopolar f.
    Cushing thumb f.
    Cushing tissue f.
    Cushing-Brown tissue f.
    Cushing-Gutsch dressing f.
    Cushing-Gutsch tissue f.
    Cushing-Taylor carbide-jaw f.
    Cushing-Vital tissue f.
    Cutler f.
    cutting f.
    cylindrical-object f.
    cystic duct f.
    cystoscopic f.
    Czerny tenaculum f.
    Dahlgren skill-cutting f.
    Dahlgren-Hudson cranial f.
    Daicoff needle-pulling f.
    Daicoff vascular f.
    Dale femoral-popliteal anastomosis f.
    Dallas lens-inserting f.
    D'Allesandro serial suture-holding f.
    Dan chalazion f.
    Dan-Gradle ciliary f.
    Danberg iris f.
    Dandy arterial f.
    Dandy hemostatic f.
    Dandy scalp hemostatic f.
    Dandy-Kolodny hemostatic f.
    Dartigues kidney-elevating f.

forceps (*continued*)

Dartigues uterine-elevating f.

Davidson pulmonary vessel f.

Davis bayonet f.

Davis capsular f.

Davis coagulating f.

Davis diathermy f.

Davis monopolar bayonet f.

Davis sterilizing f.

Davis thoracic tissue f.

Davol rongeur f.

Dawson-Yuhl rongeur f.

Dawson-Yuhl-Kerrison rongeur f.

Dawson-Yuhl-Leksell rongeur f.

De Alvarez f.

De Juan f.

Dean tonsillar f.

Dean-Shallcross tonsil-seizing f.

DeBakey aortic f.

DeBakey Autraugrip f.

DeBakey dissecting f.

DeBakey tangential occlusion f.

DeBakey thoracic f.

DeBakey tissue f.

DeBakey vascular f.

DeBakey-Bainbridge vascular f.

DeBakey-Beck multipurpose f.

DeBakey-Coloviras-Rumel thoracic f.

DeBakey-Cooley cardiovascular f.

DeBakey-Derra anastomosis f.

DeBakey-Diethrich coronary artery f.

DeBakey-Diethrich vascular f.

DeBakey-Kelly hemostatic f.

DeBakey-Liddicoat vascular f.

forceps (*continued*)

DeBakey-Mixter thoracic f.

DeBakey-Pééan cardiovascular f.

DeBakey-Rankin hemostatic f.

DeBakey-Reynolds anastomosis f.

DeBakey-Rumel thoracic f.

DeBakey-Semb f.

Decker microsurgical f.

Deddish-Potts intestinal f.

deep-surgery f.

deep-vessel f.

Defourmental f.

DeLee cervical f.

DeLee cervix-holding f.

DeLee dressing f.

DeLee obstetrical f.

DeLee ovum f.

DeLee shuttle f.

DeLee spoon tissue f.

DeLee uterine f.

DeLee uterine-packing f.

DeLee-Simpson f.

delicate thumb-dressing f.

Delrin locking-handle f.

Demarest septal f.

DeMartel appendix f.

DeMartel scalp flap f.

DeMartel-Wolfson closing f.

DeMartel-Wolfson intestinal-holding f.

Demel wire-tightening f.

Demel wire-twisting f.

Dench ear f.

Denis Browne tonsillar f.

Dennen f.

Dennis intestinal f.

dental dressing f.

depilatory dermal f.

Derf f.

DermaCare electrosurgical f.

Derra cardiovascular f.

Derra urethral f.

Derra-Cooley f.

D'Errico bayonet pituitary f.

forceps (*continued*)

D'Errico dressing f.
D'Errico hypophyseal f.
D'Errico tissue f.
Desjardins gallstone f.
Desjardins kidney pedicle f.
Desmarres chalazion f.
Desmarres lid f.
DeTakats-McKenzie brain clip-applying f.
DeVilbiss cranial f.
DeWecker f.
DeWeese axis traction obstetrical f.
Dewey obstetrical f.
Diaflex grasping f.
diathermic f.
diathermy f.
Dieffenbach f.
Diener f.
Dieter malleus f.
Diethrich right-angled hemostatic f.
dilating f.
Dingman bone-holding f.
disimpaction f.
disk f.
diskectomy f.
disposable f.
dissecting f.
dissection f.
divergent outlet f.
Dixon flamingo f.
Dixon-Lovelace hemostatic f.
Dixon-Thorpe vitreous foreign body f.
Docktor tissue f.
Dodick lens-holding f.
Dodick Nucleus Cracker f.
Dodrill f.
dolphin dissecting f.
dolphin grasping f.
dolphin-billed grasping f.
dolphin-type atraumatic f.
Donberg iris f.
donor button f.
Dorsey bayonet f.

forceps (*continued*)

double-action bone-cutting f.
double-action hump f.
double-articulated bronchoscopic f.
double-concave rat-tooth f.
double-cupped f.
double-ended needle f.
double-ended suture f.
double-ended tissue f.
double-fixation f.
double-pronged f.
double-spoon biopsy f.
Douglas ciliary f.
Douglas eye f.
Doyen gallbladder f.
Doyen intestinal f.
Doyen towel f.
Doyen uterine f.
Doyen vulsellum f.
Draeger f.
dressing f.
Drews ciliary f.
Drews intraocular f.
Drews-Sato tying f.
Dreyfus prosthesis f.
drill guide f.
duckbill f.
Duguid curved f.
dull rotation f.
dull-pointed f.
Dumont dissecting f.
Dumont jeweler's f.
Dumont Swiss dissecting f.
Dunhill f.
Duplay tenaculum f.
Duracep biopsy f.
dural f.
Duval intestinal f.
Duval lung tissue f.
Duval lung-grasping f.
Duval-Allis f.
Duval-Collin intestinal f.
Duval-Crile intestinal f.
Duval-Crile lung f.
Duval-Crile lung-grasping f.
Duval-Crile tissue f.

forceps (*continued*)
  Duval-Vital intestinal f.
  DynaBite biopsy f.
  Dyonics basket f.
  E-series bipolar f.
  ear polyp f.
  ear punch f.
  ear-dressing f.
  ear-grasping f.
  Eastman cystic duct f.
  Eber needle-holder f.
  Echlin rongeur f.
  Ecker-Kazanjian f.
  Eckhoff f.
  Eder f.
  Edna towel f.
  Effler-Groves cardiovascular
    f.
  Eisenstein hysterectomy f.
  electrocoagulating biopsy f.
  Electrosurgery f.
  electrosurgical biopsy f.
  elevating f.
  Elliott gallbladder f.
  Elliott hemostatic f.
  Elliott obstetrical f.
  Elschnig capsular f.
  Elschnig cyclodialysis f.
  Elschnig fixation f.
  Elschnig secondary
    membrane f.
  Elschnig tissue-grasping f.
  Elschnig-O'Brien fixation f.
  Elschnig-O'Brien tissue-
    grasping f.
  Elschnig-O'Connor fixation
    f.
  Emmet obstetrical f.
  end-biting f.
  Endo-Assist endoscopic f.
  Endo-therapy disposable
    biopsy f.
  endometrial polyp f.
  endoscopic biopsy f.
  endoscopic grasping f.
  endoscopic suture-cutting f.
  endospeculum f.
  endotracheal catheter f.

forceps (*continued*)
  endotracheal tube f.
  Endura dressing f.
  Englert f.
  English tissue f.
  Ennis f.
  entropion f.
  epilation f.
  episcleral f.
  Eppendorf cervical biopsy f.
  Ergo bipolar f.
  Erhardt eyelid f.
  Erich laryngeal biopsy f.
  Ernest-McDonald soft
    intraocular lens-folding f.
  Ernest-McDonald soft IOL
    folding f.
  esophageal f.
  esophagoscopic f.
  Essrig tissue f.
  ethmoid punch f.
  ethmoid-Blakesley f.
  ethmoid-cutting f.
  ethmoidal f.
  Ethridge hysterectomy f.
  Evans-Vital tissue f.
  Everett f.
  Evershears bipolar
    laparoscopic f.
  Ewald tissue f.
  Ewald-Hudson brain f.
  Ewald-Hudson dressing f.
  Ewald-Hudson tissue f.
  Ewing capsular f.
  Excel disposable biopsy f.
  exenteration f.
  exolever f.
  expansile f.
  extracapsular f.
  extracting f.
  extraction f.
  eye f.
  eye-dressing f.
  eye-fixation f.
  eyelid f.
  Förster iris f.
  Facit uterine polyp f.
  Falcao fixation f.

forceps (*continued*)
Falk lion-jaw f.
fallopian tube f.
Farabeuf bone-holding f.
Farabeuf-Lambotte bone-holding f.
Farnham nasal-cutting f.
Farrington nasal polyp f.
Farrington septal f.
Farrior wire-crimping f.
Farris tissue f.
Faure peritoneal f.
Faure uterine biopsy f.
Fauvel laryngeal f.
Fechtner conjunctiva f.
Fechtner ring f.
Fehland intestinal f.
Feilchenfeld splinter f.
fenestrated blade f.
fenestrated cup biopsy f.
fenestrated ellipsoid spiked open span biopsy f.
fenestrated spiked open span jumbo biopsy f.
Ferguson angiotribe f.
Ferguson bone-holding f.
Ferris colporrhaphy f.
Ferris Smith bone-biting f.
Ferris Smith cup rongeur f.
Ferris Smith fragment f.
Ferris Smith rongeur f.
Ferris Smith tissue f.
Ferris Smith-Kerrison f.
Ferris Smith-Spurling intervertebral disk f.
Ferris Smith-Takahashi f.
Fichman suture-cutting f.
fine arterial f.
fine dissecting f.
Fine suture-tying f.
fine tissue f.
Fine-Castroviejo suturing f.
fine-cup f.
fine-tipped up-and-down-angled bipolar f.
fine-tooth f.
Fink fixation f.
Fink tendon-tucker f.

forceps (*continued*)
Fink-Jameson oblique muscle f.
Finochietto lobectomy f.
Finochietto thoracic f.
Fischl dissecting f.
Fischmann angiotribe f.
Fish grasping f.
Fish nasal-dressing f.
Fisher advancement f.
Fisher capsular f.
Fisher iris f.
Fisher-Arlt iris f.
Fitzgerald aortic aneurysm f.
Fitzwater peanut sponge-holding f.
fixation binocular f.
fixation/anchor f.
fixed f.
flamingo antrostomy f.
Fletcher dressing f.
Fletcher sponge f.
Fletcher-Suit polyp f.
Fletcher-Van Doren sponge-holding f.
Fletcher-Van Doren uterine f.
flexible foreign body f.
flexible optical biopsy f.
fluoroscopic foreign body f.
Foerster gallbladder f.
Foerster iris f.
Foerster sponge f.
Foerster sponge-holding f.
Foerster tissue f.
Foerster uterine f.
Foerster-Ballenger f.
Foerster-Bauer sponge-holding f.
Foerster-Mueller f.
Foerster-Van Doren sponge-holding f.
Fogarty bulldog clamp-applying f.
fold f.
folding f.
Foley vas isolation f.

forceps (*continued*)
    foramen-plugging f.
    Forbes uterine-dressing f.
    f. guard
    foreign body cystoscopy f.
    foreign body eye f.
    foreign body-retrieving f.
    forward-grasping f.
    Foss cardiovascular f.
    Foss clamp f.
    Foster-Ballenger f.
    Fox bipolar electrocautery f.
    Fox tissue f.
    Fränkel cutting-tip f.
    Fränkel esophagoscopy f.
    Fränkel laryngeal f.
    Fränkel tampon f.
    fragment f.
    Francis spud chalazion f.
    Frangenheim biopsy punch
        f.
    Frangenheim hook f.
    Frankfeldt grasping f.
    Fraser f.
    Freer septal f.
    Freer-Gruenwald punch f.
    French-pattern f.
    Fricke arterial f.
    Friedman rongeur f.
    Fry nasal f.
    Fuchs capsular f.
    Fuchs capsule f.
    Fuchs capsulotomy f.
    Fuchs extracapsular f.
    Fuchs iris f.
    Fujinon biopsy f.
    Fulpit tissue f.
    Furness cornea-holding f.
    Furness polyp f.
    Gabriel Tucker f.
    galeal f.
    gall duct f.
    gallbladder f.
    gallstone f.
    Gam-Mer bone-cutting f.
    Gambale-Merrill bone-
        cutting f.
    Gardner bone f.

forceps (*continued*)
    Gardner hysterectomy f.
    Garland hysterectomy f.
    Garrigue uterine-dressing f.
    Garrison f.
    Gaskin fragment f.
    gastrointestinal f.
    Gauss hemostatic f.
    Gavin-Miller colon f.
    Gavin-Miller intestinal f.
    Gavin-Miller tissue f.
    Gaylor uterine biopsy f.
    Geissendorfer uterine f.
    Gelfilm f.
    Gelfoam pressure f.
    Gellhorn uterine biopsy f.
    Gelpi hysterectomy f.
    Gelpi-Lowrie hysterectomy
        f.
    Gemini gall duct f.
    Gemini hemostatic f.
    Gemini Mixter f.
    Gemini thoracic f.
    general tissue f.
    general wire f.
    Gerald bayonet
        microbipolar
        neurosurgical f.
    Gerald brain f.
    Gerald dressing f.
    Gerald monopolar f.
    Gerald straight microbipolar
        neurosurgical f.
    Gerald tissue f.
    Gerbode cardiovascular
        tissue f.
    GI f.
    GIA f.
    Gifford fixation f.
    Gifford iris f.
    Gilbert cystic duct f.
    Gildenberg biopsy f.
    Gill curved iris f.
    Gill incision-spreading f.
    Gill iris f.
    Gill-Arruga capsular f.
    Gill-Chandler iris f.
    Gill-Fuchs capsular f.

forceps (*continued*)
 Gill-Hess iris f.
 Gill-Safar f.
 Gill-Welsh capsular f.
 Gillespie obstetrical f.
 Gillies dissecting f.
 Gillies tissue f.
 Gillquist-Oretorp-Stille f.
 Ginsberg tissue f.
 giraffe biopsy f.
 Girard corneoscleral f.
 Glassman noncrushing
  pickup f.
 Glassman pickup f.
 Glassman-Allis intestinal f.
 Glassman-Allis noncrushing
  common duct f.
 Glassman-Allis noncrushing
  intestinal f.
 Glassman-Allis noncrushing
  tissue-holding f.
 Glassman-Babcock f.
 Glenn diverticular f.
 Glenner vaginal
  hysterectomy f.
 glenoid-reaming f.
 globular object f.
 Glover anastomosis f.
 Glover coarctation f.
 Glover curved f.
 Glover infundibular rongeur
  f.
 Glover patent ductus f.
 Glover spoon-shaped f.
 goiter vulsellum f.
 goiter-seizing f.
 Gold deep-surgery f.
 Gold hemostatic f.
 Goldman-Kazanjian nasal f.
 Goldmann capsulorrhexis f.
 Gomco f.
 Good obstetrical f.
 Goodhill tonsillar f.
 Goodyear-Gruenwald f.
 Gordon bead f.
 Gordon ciliary f.
 Gordon uterine f.
 Gordon vulsellum f.

forceps (*continued*)
 Grabow f.
 Gradle ciliary f.
 Graefe curved iris f.
 Graefe dressing f.
 Graefe eye-fixation f.
 Graefe straight iris f.
 Graefe tissue f.
 Graefe tissue-grasping f.
 Grafco-Halsted f.
 grasping biopsy f.
 grasping tripod f.
 Gray arterial f.
 Gray cystic duct f.
 Grayson corneal f.
 Grayton corneal f.
 Grazer blepharoplasty f.
 Green capsular f.
 Green chalazion f.
 Green fixation f.
 Green suction tube f.
 Green tissue-grasping f.
 Green tube-holding f.
 Green-Armytage hemostatic
  f.
 Greenwood bipolar
  coagulation-suction f.
 Gregory f.
 Greven alligator f.
 Grey Turner f.
 Grieshaber diamond-coated
  f.
 Grieshaber internal limiting
  membrane f.
 Grieshaber iris f.
 Grieshaber manipulator f.
 Griffiths-Brown f.
 grooved tying f.
 Gross dressing f.
 Gross hyoid-cutting f.
 Gross sponge f.
 Grotting f.
 Gruenwald bayonet-
  dressing f.
 Gruenwald dissecting f.
 Gruenwald dressing f.
 Gruenwald Durogrip f.
 Gruenwald ear f.

forceps (*continued*)
- Gruenwald nasal-cutting f.
- Gruenwald nasal-dressing f.
- Gruenwald tissue f.
- Gruenwald-Bryant nasal f.
- Gruenwald-Bryant nasal-cutting f.
- Gruenwald-Jansen f.
- Gruenwald-Love neurosurgical f.
- Gruppe wire-crimping f.
- Guggenheim adenoidal f.
- guide f.
- Guilford-Wright f.
- guillotome f.
- Guist fixation f.
- Gunderson bone f.
- Gunderson muscle recession f.
- Gunnar-Hey roller f.
- Guppe f.
- Gusberg uterine f.
- Gutgemann auricular appendage f.
- Gutglass hemostatic cervical f.
- Gutierrez-Najar grasping f.
- Guyton suturing f.
- Guyton-Clark f.
- Guyton-Clark fragment f.
- Guyton-Noyes fixation f.
- Haberer gastrointestinal f.
- Haberer-Gili f.
- Hagenbarth clip-applying f.
- Haig obstetrical f.
- Haig-Ferguson obstetrical f.
- Hajek antral punch f.
- Hajek-Koffler bone punch f.
- Hajek-Koffler sphenoidal f.
- Hakler f.
- Halberg contact lens f.
- Hale obstetrical f.
- Halifax placement f.
- Hallberg f.
- hallux f.
- Halsey mosquito f.
- Halsted arterial f.
- Halsted curved mosquito f.

forceps (*continued*)
- Halsted hemostatic mosquito f.
- Halsted Micro-Line arterial f.
- Halsted-Swanson tendon-passing f.
- Hamby clip-applying f.
- Hamilton deep-surgery f.
- hammer f.
- Hank-Dennen obstetrical f.
- Hannahan f.
- Hardy bayonet dressing f.
- Hardy bayonet neurosurgical bipolar f.
- Hardy microbipolar f.
- Hardy microsurgical bayonet bipolar f.
- harelip f.
- Harken cardiovascular f.
- Harken-Cooley f.
- Harman fixation f.
- Harms corneal f.
- Harms microtying f.
- Harms suture-tying f.
- Harms tying f.
- Harms utility f.
- Harms vessel f.
- Harms-Tubingen tying f.
- Harrington clamp f.
- Harrington lung-grasping f.
- Harrington thoracic f.
- Harrington vulsellum f.
- Harrington-Mayo tissue f.
- Harrington-Mixter thoracic f.
- Harris suture-carrying f.
- Harrison bone-holding f.
- Hartmann alligator f.
- Hartmann ear polyp f.
- Hartmann ear-dressing f.
- Hartmann hemostatic mosquito f.
- Hartmann mosquito hemostatic f.
- Hartmann nasal polyp f.
- Hartmann nasal-cutting f.
- Hartmann nasal-dressing f.
- Hartmann tonsillar punch f.

forceps (*continued*)

Hartmann uterine biopsy f.
Hartmann-Citelli alligator f.
Hartmann-Citelli ear punch f.
Hartmann-Corgill ear f.
Hartmann-Gruenwald nasal-cutting f.
Hartmann-Herzfeld ear f.
Hartmann-Noyes nasal-dressing f.
Hartmann-Proctor ear f.
Hartmann-Weingärtner ear f.
Hartmann-Wullstein ear f.
Haslinger tip f.
Hasner lid f.
Hasson bullet-tip f.
Hasson grasping f.
Hasson needle-nose f.
Hasson ring f.
Hasson spike-tooth f.
Haugh ear f.
Hawkins cervical biopsy f.
Hawks-Dennen obstetrical f.
Hayes anterior resection f.
Hayes Martin f.
Hayes-Olivecrona f.
Hayton-Williams f.
Healy gastrointestinal f.
Healy intestinal f.
Healy suture-removing f.
Healy uterine biopsy f.
Heaney hysterectomy f.
Heaney tissue f.
Heaney-Kantor hysterectomy f.
Heaney-Rezek f.
Heaney-Simon hysterectomy f.
Heaney-Stumf f.
Heath chalazion f.
Heath clip-removing f.
Heath nasal f.
Hecht fascia lata f.
Heermann alligator f.
Heermann ear f.

forceps (*continued*)

Hegenbarth clip-applying f.
Hegenbarth-Michel clip-applying f.
Heidelberg fixation f.
Heifitz cup serrated ring f.
Heiming kidney stone f.
Heiss arterial f.
Heiss hemostatic f.
Heiss vulsellum f.
Heller biopsy f.
Hemoclip-applying f.
hemorrhoidal f.
hemostatic cervical f.
hemostatic clip-applying f.
hemostatic neurosurgical f.
hemostatic tissue f.
hemostatic tonsillar f.
hemostatic tracheal f.
Hendren cardiovascular f.
Hendren pediatric f.
Henke punch f.
Henrotin vulsellum f.
Henry ciliary f.
Herff membrane-puncturing f.
Herget biopsy f.
Hermann bone-holding f.
Herrick kidney f.
Hersh LASIK retreatment f.
Hertel kidney stone f.
Hertel rigid dilator stone f.
Hertel rigid kidney stone f.
Herz meniscal tendon f.
Herzfeld ear f.
Hess capsular f.
Hess iris f.
Hess-Barraquer iris f.
Hess-Gill iris f.
Hess-Horwitz iris f.
Hessburg lens-inserting f.
Hevesy polyp f.
Heyman nasal f.
Heyman nasal-cutting f.
Heyman-Knight nasal dressing f.
Heyner f.
Heywood-Smith dressing f.

forceps (*continued*)

Heywood-Smith gallbladder f.

Heywood-Smith sponge-holding f.

Hibbs biting f.

Hibbs bone-cutting f.

Hibbs bone-holding f.

Hildebrandt uterine hemostatic f.

Hildyard nasal f.

Himalaya dressing f.

Hinderer cartilage f.

Hirsch hypophysis punch f.

Hirschman hemorrhoidal f.

Hirschman jeweler's f.

Hirschman lens f.

Hirst obstetrical f.

Hirst placental f.

Hirst-Emmet obstetrical f.

Hirst-Emmet placental f.

Hodge obstetrical f.

Hoen alligator f.

Hoen bayonet f.

Hoen dressing f.

Hoen grasping f.

Hoen hemostatic f.

Hoen scalp f.

Hoen tissue f.

Hoffmann ear punch f.

Hoffmann-Pollock f.

holding f.

Holinger specimen f.

hollow-object f.

Holmes fixation f.

Holth punch f.

Holzbach hysterectomy f.

hook f.

Hopkins aortic f.

Horsley bone-cutting f.

Horsley-Stille bone-cutting f.

Horsley-Stille rib shears f.

Hosemann choledochus f.

Hosford-Hicks transfer f.

Hoskins beaked Colibri f.

Hoskins fine straight f.

Hoskins fixation f.

Hoskins microstraight f.

forceps (*continued*)

Hoskins miniaturized micro straight f.

Hoskins straight microiris f.

Hoskins suture f.

Hoskins-Dallas intraocular lens-inserting f.

Hoskins-Luntz f.

Hoskins-Skeleton fine f.

Hoskins-Skeleton grooved broad-tipped f.

host tissue f.

hot biopsy f.

hot flexible f.

hot Sampler disposable hot biopsy f.

House alligator crimper f.

House alligator grasping f.

House alligator strut f.

House cup f.

House ear f.

House Gelfoam pressure f.

House grasping f.

House miniature f.

House oval-cup f.

House pressure f.

House strut f.

House-Dieter eye f.

House-Wullstein cup ear f.

Housepian clip-applying f.

Houspian clip-applying f.

Howard closing f.

Howard tonsil-ligating f.

Howard tonsillar f.

Howmedica Microfixation System f.

Hoxworth f.

Hoyt deep-surgery f.

Hoyt hemostatic f.

Hoytenberger tissue f.

Hubbard corneoscleral f.

Huber f. handle

Hudson brain f.

Hudson cranial f.

Hudson dressing f.

Hudson rongeur f.

Hudson tissue f.

Hufnagel mitral valve f.

forceps (*continued*)
Hulka clip f.
Hulka tenaculum f.
Hulka-Kenwick uterine-
elevating f.
Hulka-Kenwick uterine-
manipulating f.
hump f.
Hunt angled serrated ring f.
Hunt angled-tip f.
Hunt bipolar f.
Hunt chalazion f.
Hunt grasping f.
Hunt tumor f.
Hunt vessel f.
Hunt-Yasargil pituitary f.
Hunter splinter f.
Hurd bone f.
Hurd bone-cutting f.
Hurd septal bone-
cutting f.
Hurd septum-cutting f.
Hurdner tissue f.
Hurteau f.
Hyde double-curved
corneal f.
hyoid-cutting f.
hypogastric artery f.
hypophyseal f.
hypophysectomy f.
hysterectomy f.
I-tech intraocular foreign
body f.
I-tech splinter f.
I-tech tying f.
Ilg capsular f.
Ilg curved micro tying f.
Ilg insertion f.
iliac f.
Iliff blepharochalasis f.
IM Jaws alligator f.
Imperatori laryngeal f.
implant f.
implantation f.
Inamura small incision
capsulorrhexis f.
infant biopsy f.
infundibular f.

forceps (*continued*)
Ingraham-Fowler clip-
applying f.
inlet f.
insertion f.
instrument-grasping f.
insulated bayonet f.
insulated monopolar f.
insulated tissue f.
intervertebral disk f.
intestinal anastomosis f.
intestinal closing f.
intestinal holding f.
intestinal tissue f.
intracapsular lens f.
intraocular irrigating f.
intraocular lens f.
intrathoracic f.
introducing f.
Iowa membrane f.
Iowa State fixation f.
Iowa-Mengert membrane f.
iris bipolar f.
iris tissue f.
Iselin f.
isolation f.
Jackson alligator grasping f.
Jackson approximation f.
Jackson biopsy f.
Jackson broad staple f.
Jackson button f.
Jackson conventional
foreign body f.
Jackson cross-action f.
Jackson cylindrical-object f.
Jackson double-concave
rat-tooth f.
Jackson double-prong f.
Jackson down-jaw f.
Jackson dressing f.
Jackson dull rotation f.
Jackson dull-pointed f.
Jackson endoscopic f.
Jackson fenestrated
peanut-grasping f.
Jackson flexible upper lobe
bronchus f.
Jackson forward-grasping f.

forceps (*continued*)
  Jackson globular object f.
  Jackson head-holding f.
  Jackson hemostatic f.
  Jackson hollow-object f.
  Jackson infant biopsy f.
  Jackson laryngeal
    applicator f.
  Jackson laryngeal basket f.
  Jackson laryngeal punch f.
  Jackson laryngeal ring-
    rotation f.
  Jackson laryngeal-dressing f.
  Jackson laryngeal-grasping f.
  Jackson laryngofissure f.
  Jackson papilloma f.
  Jackson pin-bending
    costophrenic f.
  Jackson punch f.
  Jackson ring-jaw f.
  Jackson ring-rotation f.
  Jackson sharp-pointed
    rotation f.
  Jackson side-curved f.
  Jackson sister-hook f.
  Jackson tendon-seizing f.
  Jackson tracheal
    hemostatic f.
  Jackson triangular-punch f.
  Jacob capsule fragment f.
  Jacobs biopsy f.
  Jacobs capsular fragment f.
  Jacobs vulsellum f.
  Jacobson bipolar f.
  Jacobson dressing f.
  Jacobson hemostatic f.
  Jacobson mosquito f.
  Jaffe capsulorhexis f.
  Jaffe suturing f.
  Jager meniscal f.
  Jako laryngeal f.
  Jako microlaryngeal cup f.
  Jako microlaryngeal
    grasping f.
  James wound-
    approximation f.
  Jameson muscle recession
    f.

forceps (*continued*)
  Jameson strabismus f.
  Jameson tracheal muscle f.
  Jannetta alligator grasping f.
  Jannetta bayonet f.
  Jannetta microbayonet f.
  Jansen bayonet dressing f.
  Jansen bayonet ear f.
  Jansen bayonet nasal f.
  Jansen dissecting f.
  Jansen dressing f.
  Jansen monopolar f.
  Jansen nasal-dressing f.
  Jansen thumb f.
  Jansen-Gruenwald f.
  Jansen-Middleton nasal-
    cutting f.
  Jansen-Middleton punch f.
  Jansen-Middleton septal f.
  Jansen-Middleton
    septotomy f.
  Jansen-Middleton septum-
    cutting f.
  Jansen-Mueller f.
  Jansen-Struyken septal f.
  Jarcho tenaculum f.
  Jarell f.
  Jarit brain f.
  Jarit microsuture tying f.
  Jarit mosquito f.
  Jarit sterilizer f.
  Jarit tendon-pulling f.
  Jarit tube-occluding f.
  Jarit wire-pulling f.
  Jarit-Allis tissue f.
  Jarit-Crafoord f.
  Jarit-Dandy f.
  Jarit-Liston bone-cutting f.
  Jarvis hemorrhoidal f.
  Javerts placental f.
  Javerts polyp f.
  Jayles f.
  Jensen intraocular lens f.
  Jensen lens-inserting f.
  Jerald f.
  Jervey capsular fragment f.
  Jervey iris f.
  Jesberg grasping f.

forceps (*continued*)
  jeweler's bipolar f.
  jeweler's pickup f.
  John Weiss f.
  Johns Hopkins gall duct f.
  Johns Hopkins gallbladder
    f.
  Johns Hopkins hemostatic
    f.
  Johns Hopkins occluding f.
  Johns Hopkins serrefine f.
  Johnson brain tumor f.
  Johnson ptosis f.
  Johnson thoracic f.
  Jones hemostatic f.
  Jones IMA f.
  Jones towel f.
  Joplin bone-holding f.
  Jordan strut f.
  Judd strabismus f.
  Judd suture f.
  Judd-Allis intestinal f.
  Judd-Allis tissue f.
  Judd-DeMartel gallbladder
    f.
  Juers crimper f.
  Juers lingual f.
  Juers-Lempert rongeur f.
  jugum f.
  Julian splenorenal f.
  Julian thoracic artery f.
  Julian-Damian thoracic f.
  jumbo f.
  Jurasz laryngeal f.
  Küstner uterine tenaculum
    f.
  K/S-Allis f.
  Kadesky f.
  Kahler bronchial biopsy f.
  Kahler bronchoscopic f.
  Kahler bronchus-grasping f.
  Kahler laryngeal biopsy f.
  Kahler polyp f.
  Kahn tenaculum f.
  Kalman occluding f.
  Kalman tube-occluding f.
  Kalt capsular f.
  Kansas University corneal f.

forceps (*continued*)
  Kantor f.
  Kantrowitz dressing f.
  Kantrowitz thoracic f.
  Kantrowitz tissue f.
  Kapp f.
  Kapp-Beck f.
  Karl Storz reusable multi-
    function valve trocar take-
    apart scissors f.
  Karp aortic punch f.
  Katena f.
  Katzin-Barraquer Colibri f.
  Katzin-Barraquer corneal f.
  Kaufman ENT f.
  Kazanjian bone-cutting f.
  Kazanjian cutting f.
  Kazanjian nasal f.
  Kazanjian nasal hump f.
  Kazanjian-Cottle f.
  Keeler extended round tip
    f.
  Keeler intraocular foreign
    body grasping f.
  Keen Edge disposable
    biopsy f.
  Kelly arterial f.
  Kelly dressing f.
  Kelly hemostatic f.
  Kelly ovum f.
  Kelly placental f.
  Kelly polypus f.
  Kelly tissue f.
  Kelly urethral f.
  Kelly-Gray uterine f.
  Kelly-Murphy f.
  Kelly-Rankin f.
  Kelman implantation f.
  Kelman intraocular f.
  Kelman irrigator f.
  Kelman-McPherson corneal
    f.
  Kelman-McPherson
    microtying f.
  Kelman-McPherson suture
    f.
  Kelman-McPherson tissue f.
  Kelman-McPherson tying f.

forceps (*continued*)
    Kennedy vulsellum f.
    Kennerdell bayonet f.
    Kent f.
    keratotomy f.
    Kern bone-holding f.
    Kern-Lane bone-holding f.
    Kerrison f.
    Kershner one-step micro
        capsulorhexis f.
    Kevorkian uterine biopsy f.
    Kevorkian-Younge cervical
        biopsy f.
    Kevorkian-Younge uterine
        biopsy f.
    Khodadad microclip f.
    kidney pedicle f.
    kidney stone f.
    kidney-elevating f.
    Kielland f.
    Killian septal compression
        f.
    Killian-Jameson f.
    Kinder Design pedo f.
    King tissue f.
    King wound f.
    King-Prince muscle f.
    King-Prince recession f.
    Kingsley grasping f.
    Kirby capsular f.
    Kirby corneoscleral f.
    Kirby eye tissue f.
    Kirby fixation f.
    Kirby intracapsular lens f.
    Kirby iris f.
    Kirby lens f.
    Kirby-Arthus fixation f.
    Kirby-Bracken iris f.
    Kirkpatrick tonsillar f.
    Kirschner-Ullrich f.
    Kirwan bipolar
        electrosurgical f.
    Kirwan coaptation
        ophthalmic bipolar f.
    Kirwan iris curved
        ophthalmic bipolar f.
    Kirwan iris straight
        ophthalmic bipolar f.

forceps (*continued*)
    Kirwan jeweler's curved
        ophthalmic bipolar f.
    Kirwan jeweler's insulated
        straight ophthalmic
        bipolar f.
    Kirwan-Adson ophthalmic
        bipolar f.
    Kirwan-Nadler-style
        coaptation ophthalmic
        bipolar f.
    Kirwan-Tenzel ophthalmic
        bipolar f.
    Kitner goiter f.
    Kitner thyroid-packing f.
    Kjelland obstetrical f.
    Kjelland-Barton f.
    Kjelland-Luikart obstetrical
        f.
    KleenSpec f.
    Kleinert-Kutz bone-cutting f.
    Kleinert-Kutz rongeur f.
    Kleinert-Kutz tendon f.
    Kleinert-Kutz tendon-
        passing f.
    Kleinert-Kutz tendon-
        retrieving f.
    Kleppinger bipolar f.
    KLI bipolar f.
    KLI monopolar f.
    Knapp trachoma f.
    Knapp-Luer trachoma f.
    Knight nasal septum-cutting
        f.
    Knight nasal-cutting f.
    Knight polyp f.
    Knight septal f.
    Knight septum-cutting f.
    Knight turbinate f.
    Knight-Sluder nasal f.
    Knighton-Crawford f.
    Knolle lens implantation f.
    Knolle-Shepard lens f.
    Knolle-Volker lens-holding
        f.
    knot-holding f.
    knotting f.
    Koby cataract f.

forceps (*continued*)
    Kocher arterial f.
    Kocher artery f.
    Kocher hemostatic f.
    Kocher kidney-elevating f.
    Kocher Micro-Line
      intestinal f.
    Kocher-Ochsner hemostatic
      f.
    Koeberlé f.
    Koenig vascular f.
    Koerte gallstone f.
    Koffler septal f.
    Koffler-Lillie septal f.
    Kogan endospeculum f.
    Kolb bronchial f.
    Kolodny f.
    Korte gallstone f.
    Kos crimper f.
    Krönlein hemostatic f.
    Kraff intraocular utility f.
    Kraff lens-inserting f.
    Kraff suturing f.
    Kraff tying f.
    Kraff-Osher lens f.
    Kraff-Utrata capsulorrhexis
      f.
    Kraff-Utrata intraocular
      utility f.
    Kraff-Utrata tear
      capsulotomy f.
    Kramer f.
    Kratz lens-inserting f.
    Krause biopsy f.
    Krause esophagoscopy f.
    Krause punch f.
    Krause Universal f.
    Kremer fixation f.
    Kremer two-point fixation f.
    Kronfeld micropin f.
    Kronfeld suturing f.
    Krukenberg pigment
      spindle f.
    Kuhne coverglass f.
    Kuhnt capsular f.
    Kuhnt capsule f.
    Kuhnt fixation f.
    Kulvin-Kalt iris f.

forceps (*continued*)
    Kurze microbiopsy f.
    Kurze micrograsping f.
    Kurze pickup f.
    Kwapis interdental f.
    Löw-Beer f.
    Löwenberg f.
    Laborde f.
    Lahey arterial f.
    Lahey dissecting f.
    Lahey gall duct f.
    Lahey goiter vulsellum f.
    Lahey goiter-seizing f.
    Lahey hemostatic f.
    Lahey lock arterial f.
    Lahey thoracic f.
    Lahey thyroid tenaculum f.
    Lahey thyroid tissue
      traction f.
    Lahey thyroid traction
      vulsellum f.
    Lahey-Babcock f.
    Lahey-Péan f.
    Lahey-Sweet dissecting f.
    Lajeune hemostatic f.
    Lalonde delicate hook f.
    Lalonde extra fine skin
      hook f.
    Lambert chalazion f.
    Lambert-Kay anastomosis f.
    Lambotte bone-holding f.
    Lambotte fibular f.
    Lancaster-O'Connor f.
    lancet-shaped biopsy f.
    Landers vitrectomy lens f.
    Landolt spreading f.
    Landon f.
    Lane bone-holding f.
    Lane gastrointestinal f.
    Lane intestinal f.
    Lane screw-holding f.
    Lane tissue f.
    Lang iris f.
    Lange approximation f.
    Langenbeck bone-holding f.
    laparoscopic f.
    Laplace f.
    large-angled f.

forceps (*continued*)
> LaRoe undermining f.
> Larsen tendon f.
> Larsen tendon-holding f.
> laryngeal applicator f.
> laryngeal basket f.
> laryngeal biopsy f.
> laryngeal bronchial
>   grasping f.
> laryngeal curette f.
> laryngeal grasping f.
> laryngeal punch f.
> laryngeal rotation f.
> laryngeal sponging f.
> laryngofissure f.
> laser microlaryngeal cup f.
> laser microlaryngeal
>   grasping f.
> laser ovary f.
> Laufe divergent outlet f.
> Laufe obstetrical f.
> Laufe uterine polyp f.
> Laufe-Barton obstetrical f.
> Laufe-Barton-Kjelland
>   obstetrical f.
> Laufe-Barton-Kjelland-Piper
>   obstetrical f.
> Laufe-Piper obstetrical f.
> Laufe-Piper uterine polyp f.
> Laufman f.
> Laurer f.
> Laval advancement f.
> Lawrence deep f.
> Lawrence hemostatic f.
> Lawton f.
> Lawton-Schubert biopsy f.
> Lawton-Wittner cervical
>   biopsy f.
> Lazar microsuction f.
> Leader vas isolation f.
> Leahey chalazion f.
> Leahey marginal chalazion
>   f.
> Leahey suture f.
> Leasure nasal f.
> Leaver sclerotomy f.
> Lebsche f.
> Lees arterial f.

forceps (*continued*)
> Lees nontraumatic f.
> Lefferts bone-cutting f.
> Leibinger Micro System
>   plate-holding f.
> Leigh capsular f.
> Lejeune thoracic f.
> Leksell rongeur f.
> Leland-Jones f.
> Lemmon-Russian f.
> Lemoine f.
> Lempert rongeur f.
> lens implantation f.
> lens loop f.
> lens-threading f.
> Leo Schwartz sponge-
>   holding f.
> Leonard f.
> Leriche hemostatic f.
> Leriche tissue f.
> LeRoy clip-applying f.
> Lester fixation f.
> Lester muscle f.
> Levenson tissue f.
> Levora fixation f.
> Levret f.
> Lewin bone-holding f.
> Lewin spinal-perforating f.
> Lewis septal f.
> Lewis tonsillar hemostatic f.
> Lewis ureteral stone
>   isolation f.
> Lewkowitz lithotomy f.
> Lewkowitz ovum f.
> Lewkowitz placental f.
> Lexer tissue f.
> Leyro-Diaz thoracic f.
> lid f.
> Lieb-Guerry f.
> Lieberman suturing f.
> Lieberman tying f.
> Lieberman-Pollock double
>   corneal f.
> ligament-grasping f.
> ligamentum flavum f.
> ligature f.
> ligature-carrying f.
> Lillehei valve-grasping f.

forceps (*continued*)
Lillie intestinal f.
Lillie tissue-holding f.
Lillie-Killian septal f.
Lindsay-Rea f.
Lindstrom lens-insertion f.
lingual f.
Linn-Graefe iris f.
Linnartz f.
lion f.
lion-jaw bone-holding f.
Lister conjunctival f.
Liston bone-cutting f.
Liston-Key bone-cutting f.
Liston-Key-Horsley f.
Liston-Littauer bone-cutting
f.
Liston-Stille bone-cutting f.
lithotomy f.
Litt f.
Littauer bone-cutting f.
Littauer ciliary f.
Littauer ear polyp f.
Littauer ear-dressing f.
Littauer nasal-dressing f.
Littauer-Liston bone-cutting
f.
Littauer-West cutting f.
Littlewood tissue f.
Livernois lens-holding f.
Livernois pickup and
folding f.
Livingston f.
Llobera fixation f.
Llorente dissecting f.
Lloyd-Davies occlusion f.
lobe-grasping f.
lobe-holding f.
lobectomy f.
Lobell splinter f.
Lobenstein-Tarnier f.
lobster bone-reduction f.
Lockwood intestinal f.
Lockwood tissue f.
Lockwood-Allis intestinal f.
Lockwood-Allis tissue f.
Lombard-Beyer f.
London tissue f.

forceps (*continued*)
Long Island College
Hospital placental f.
long tissue f.
long-jaw basket f.
loop-type snare f.
loop-type stone-crushing f.
loose body suction f.
Lordan chalazion f.
Lore subglottic f.
Lore suction tube and tip-
holding f.
Lore suction tube-holding f.
Lothrop ligature f.
Love-Gruenwald alligator f.
Love-Gruenwald pituitary f.
Love-Kerrison rongeur f.
Lovelace bladder f.
Lovelace gallbladder
traction f.
Lovelace hemostatic f.
Lovelace lung-grasping f.
Lovelace thyroid-traction
vulsellum f.
Lovelace tissue f.
Lovelace traction lung f.
Lovelace traction tissue f.
low outlet f.
lower gall duct f.
lower lateral f.
Lowis intervertebral disk f.
Lowman bone-holding f.
Lowsley grasping f.
Lowsley prostatic f.
Lowsley-Luc f.
Luc ethmoidal f.
Luc f.
Luc nasal-cutting f.
Luc septal f.
Luc septum-cutting f.
Lucae bayonet dressing f.
Lucae bayonet ear f.
Lucae bayonet tissue f.
Lucae dissecting f.
Lucae ear f.
Luer curette f.
Luer hemorrhoidal f.
Luer rongeur f.

forceps (*continued*)
Luer-Whiting f.
Luer-Whiting rongeur f.
Luhr Microfixation System
plate-holding f.
Luikart f.
Luikart-Bill f.
Luikart-Kjelland obstetrical f.
Luikart-McLane obstetrical f.
Luikart-Simpson obstetrical
f.
lung tissue f.
lung-grasping f.
Lutz septal f.
Lynch cup-shaped curette f.
Lynch laryngeal f.
Lyon f.
McCain TMJ f.
McCarthy visual hemostatic
f.
McCarthy-Alcock f.
MacCarty f.
McClintock placental f.
McClintock uterine f.
MacGregor conjunctival f.
McCollough tying f.
McCoy septal f.
McCoy septum-cutting f.
McCullough strabismus f.
McCullough suture-tying f.
McCullough suturing f.
McDonald lens-folding f.
McGannon lens f.
McGee wire-closure f.
McGee wire-crimping f.
McGee-Paparella wire-
crimping f.
McGee-Priest wire f.
McGee-Priest wire-closure
f.
McGee-Priest-Paparella f.
McGill f.
McGivney hemorrhoidal f.
McGravey tissue f.
McGregor conjunctival f.
McGuire marginal chalazion
f.
McHenry tonsillar f.

forceps (*continued*)
McIndoe bone-cutting f.
McIndoe dissecting f.
McIndoe dressing f.
McIndoe rongeur f.
McIntosh suture-holding f.
McKay ear f.
MacKenty tissue f.
McKenzie clip-applying f.
McKernan f.
McKernan-Adson f.
McKernan-Potts f.
McLane obstetrical f.
McLane pile f.
McLane-Luikart obstetrical
f.
McLane-Tucker obstetrical
f.
McLane-Tucker-Kjelland f.
McLane-Tucker-Luikart f.
McLean capsular f.
McLean muscle-recession f.
McLean ophthalmic f.
McLearie bone f.
McNealey-Glassman-Mixter
f.
McNealy-Glassman-
Babcock f.
McPherson angled f.
McPherson bent f.
McPherson corneal f.
McPherson irrigating f.
McPherson lens f.
McPherson microbipolar f.
McPherson microcorneal f.
McPherson microiris f.
McPherson microsuture f.
McPherson straight bipolar
f.
McPherson suture-tying f.
McPherson tying iris f.
McPherson-Castroviejo f.
McPherson-Pierse
microcorneal f.
McPherson-Pierse
microsuturing f.
McQueen vitreous f.
McQuigg f.

forceps (*continued*)

McQuigg-Mixter bronchial f.
McWhorter tonsillar f.
Machemer diamond-dust-coated foreign body f.
Machemer diamond-dusted f.
Madden f.
Madden-Potts intestinal f.
Madden-Potts tissue f.
Magielski coagulating f.
Magielski tonsil-seizing f.
Magielski tonsillar f.
Magielski-Heermann strut f.
Magill catheter f.
Magill endotracheal f.
Maier dressing f.
Maier polyp f.
Maier sponge f.
Maier uterine f.
Mailler colon f.
Mailler cut-off f.
Mailler intestinal f.
Mailler rectal f.
Maingot hysterectomy f.
Malis angled bayonet f.
Malis bipolar coagulation f.
Malis bipolar cutting f.
Malis bipolar irrigating f.
Malis cup f.
Malis jeweler bipolar f.
Malis titanium microsurgical f.
Malis-Jensen bipolar f.
Malis-Jensen microbipolar f.
malleus f.
mammary-coronary tissue f.
Manche LASIK f.
Manhattan Eye Ear suturing f.
Mann f.
Manning f.
Mansfield f.
Mantis retrograde f.
March-Barton f.
Marcuse f.
marginal chalazion f.
Markwalder rib f.

forceps (*continued*)

Marshik tonsil-seizing f.
Marshik tonsillar f.
Martin bipolar coagulation f.
Martin cartilage f.
Martin meniscal f.
Martin nasopharyngeal biopsy f.
Martin nasopharyngeal f.
Martin thumb f.
Martin tissue f.
Martin uterine tenaculum f.
Maryan biopsy punch f.
Masket f.
Masterson hysterectomy f.
Mastin goiter f.
Mastin muscle f.
Mathieu foreign body f.
Mathieu tongue f.
Mathieu urethral f.
matte black f.
Matthew f.
Maumenee capsular f.
Maumenee corneal f.
Maumenee cross-action capsular f.
Maumenee straight-action capsular f.
Maumenee Suregrip f.
Maumenee tissue f.
Maumenee-Colibri corneal f.
Max Fine tying f.
maxillary disimpaction f.
maxillary fracture f.
Maxum Carr-Locke angled f.
Maxum reusable endoscopic f.
Mayer f.
Mayfield aneurysm f.
Mayo bone-cutting f.
Mayo kidney pedicle f.
Mayo tissue f.
Mayo ureter isolation f.
Mayo-Harrington f.
Mayo-Ochsner f.
Mayo-Robson gastrointestinal f.

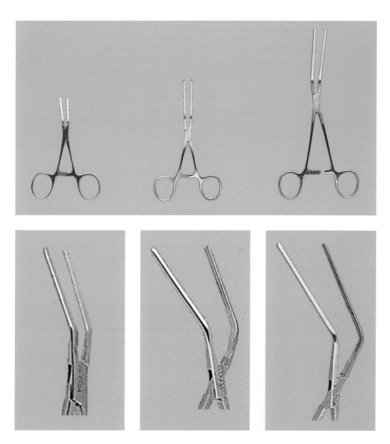

Left to right, 2 pediatric bulldog clamps: front view, tip; 2 DeBakey bulldog clamps: front view, tip; 2 DeBakey peripheral vascular clamps, front view, tip.

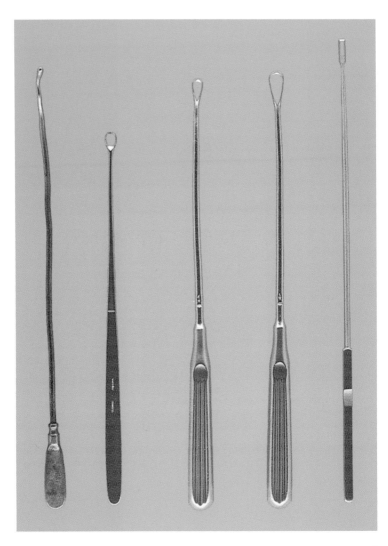

Left to right, 1 Sims uterine sound; 1 Heaney uterine curette, sharp, serrated tip; 1 Thomas uterine curette semirigid, dull, small; 1 Sims uterine curette semirigid, sharp, medium; 1 Kevorkian curette.

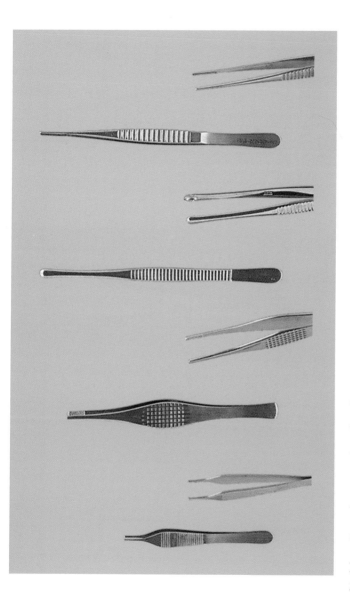

Left to right, Adson tissue forceps and tip; Ferris-Smith tissue forceps and tip; Russian tissue forceps and tip; DeBakey Autraugrip tissue forceps and tip.

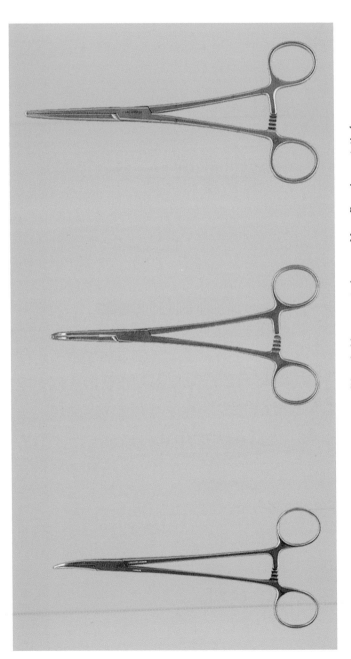

Left to right, Tonsil hemostatic forceps; Westphal hemostatic forceps; Mayo Pean hemostatic forceps.

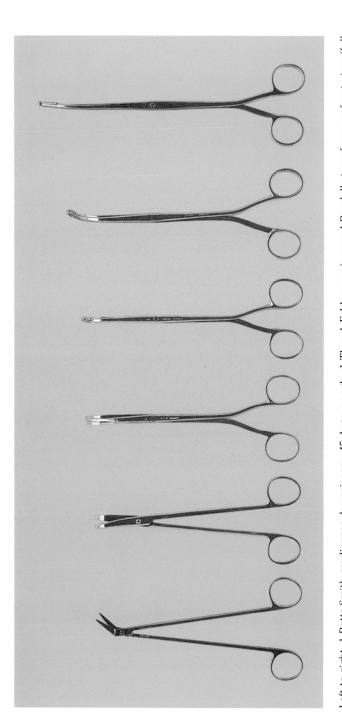

Left to right, 1 Potts-Smith cardiovascular scissors, 45-degree angle; 1 Thorek-Feldman scissors; 4 Randall stone forceps, front view (full curved, ¾ curved, ½ curved and ¼ curved).

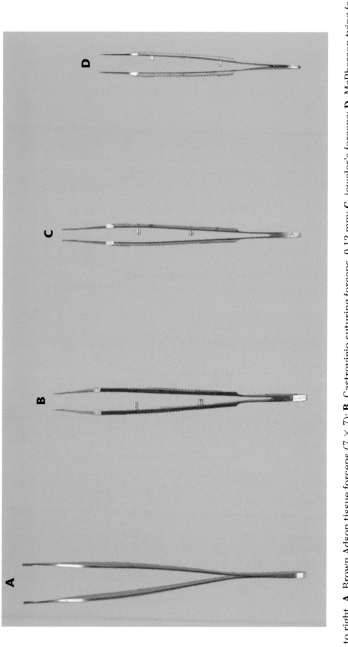

Left to right, **A**, Brown Adson tissue forceps (7 × 7); **B**, Castroviejo suturing forceps, 0.12 mm; **C**, jeweler's forceps; **D**, McPherson tying forceps, straight.

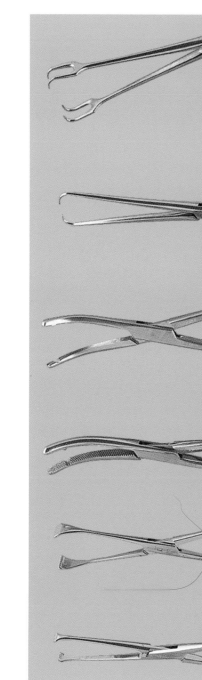

Left to right, Tips: 1 Allis tissue forceps; 1 Allis-Adair tissue forceps; 1 Heaney hysterectomy forceps; 1 Ballentine Heaney hysterectomy forceps; 1 Schroeder uterine tenaculum forceps, single tooth; 1 Skene uterine vulsellum forceps, double tooth, straight.

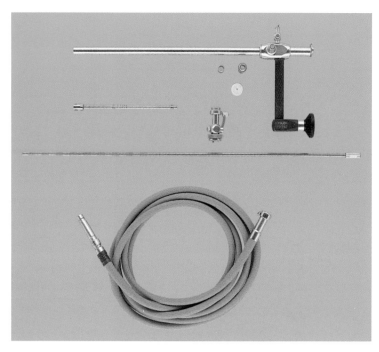

Top to bottom, Laparoscope and fiberoptic light cord.

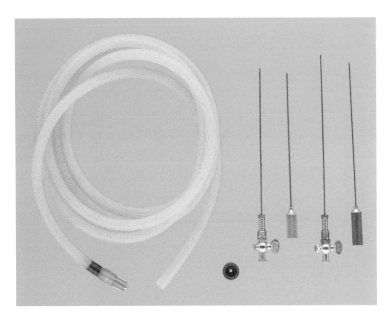

Left to right, 1 Silastic tubing, 8 foot long, with one male Luer-Lok end; 1 rubber cap; 1 Verres needle stylet, medium; 1 Verres needle, medium; 1 Verres needle stylet, long; 1 Verres needle, long.

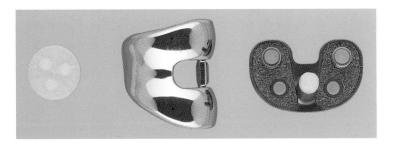

Nex Gen system. Left to right, 1 patella button; 1 femoral component; 1 porous stem-tibial base plate.

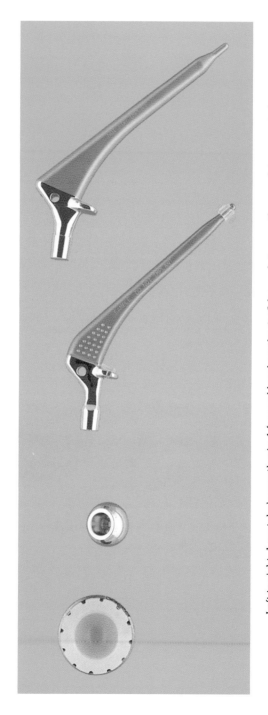

Left to right, 1 acetabular prothesis; 1 femoral head prothesis; 2 femoral stem protheses: plain, cemented.

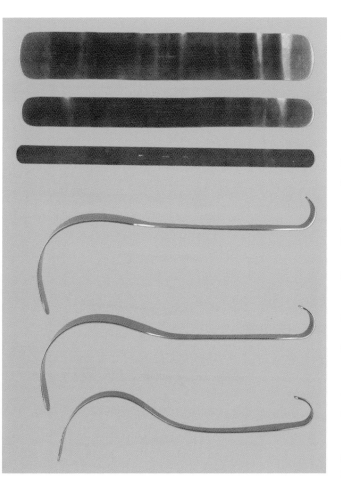

Left to right, Deaver retractors, small, medium, and large; Ochsner malleable retractors, narrow, medium, and wide.

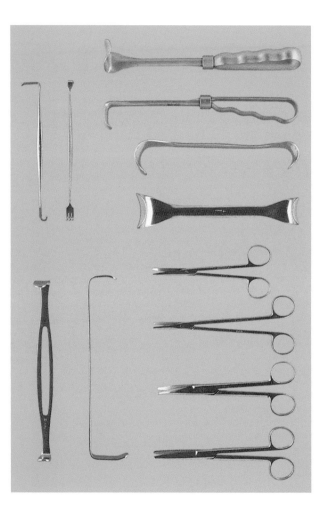

Top pairs, left to right, 2 Army Navy retractors, front view, side view; 2 Miller-Senn retractors, side view, front view. Bottom, left to right, 2 Mayo dissecting scissors, straight, curved; 2 Metzenbaum dissecting scissors, 7 inch, 5 inch; 2 Goelet retractors, front view, side view; 2 Richardson retractors, small.

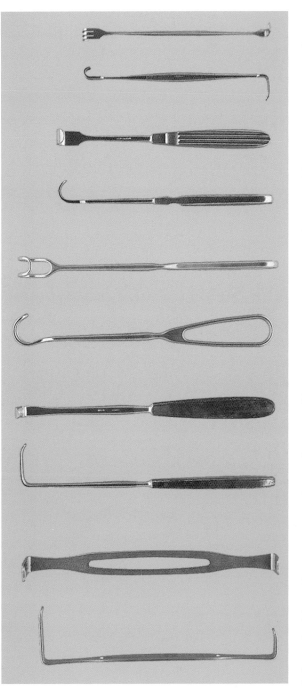

Left to right, 2 Army Navy retractors, side view, front view; 2 Langenbeck retractors, side view, front view; 2 Green goiter retractors, side view, front view; 2 Cushing vein retractors, side view, front view; 2 Miller-Senn retractors, side view, front view.

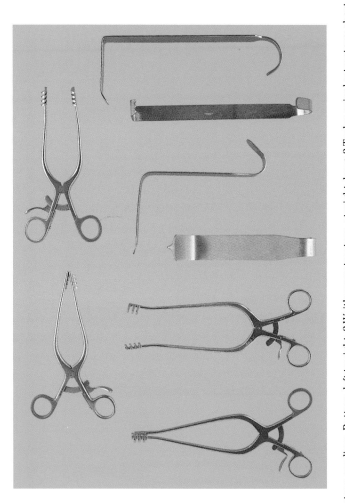

Top, 2 Adson retractors, medium. Bottom, left to right, 2 Weitlaner retractors, straight, long; 2 Taylor spinal retractors: short, front view; long, side view; 2 Hibbs laminectomy retractors: narrow, front view; wide, side view.

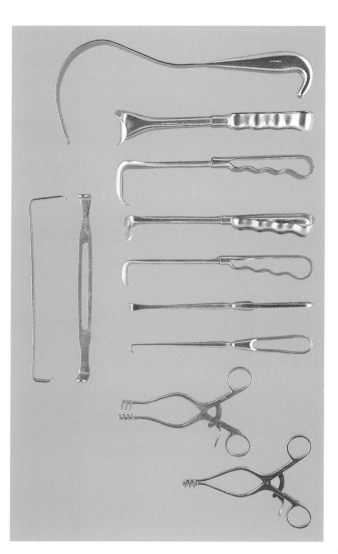

Top, 2 Army Navy retractors, side view, front view. Bottom, left to right, 2 Weitlaner retractors, sharp, medium; 2 vein retractors, side view, front view; 4 Richardson retractors, 2 small, 2 medium; 1 Deaver retractors, small.

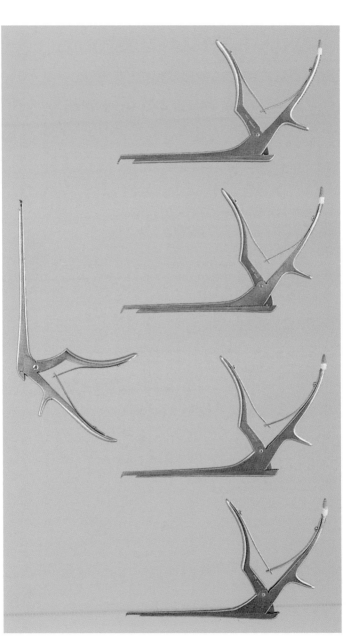

Top, 1 Kerrison rongeur, 45 degree, 1 mm. Bottom, left ro right, 4 Kerrison rongeurs, 45 degree, 2, 3, 4, and 5 mm.

forceps (*continued*)
    Mayo-Russian
      gastrointestinal f.
    Mazzariello-Caprini stone f.
    Mazzocco flexible lens f.
    Meacham-Scoville f.
    meat f.
    meat-grasping f.
    mechanical finger f.
    Medicon wire-twister f.
    Medicon-Jackson rectal f.
    Medicon-Packer mosquito
      f.
    medium f.
    Meeker deep-surgery f.
    Meeker gallbladder f.
    Meeker hemostatic f.
    Meeker intestinal f.
    meibomian expressor f.
    membrane f.
    membrane-puncturing f.
    Mendel ligature f.
    Mendez multi-purpose
      LASIK f.
    Mengert membrane-
      puncturing f.
    meniscal basket f.
    Mentor-Maumenee Suregrip
      f.
    Merlin stone f.
    Merriam f.
    Merz hysterectomy f.
    Metico f.
    Metzel-Wittmoser f.
    Metzenbaum tonsillar f.
    Metzenbaum-Tydings f.
    MGH uterine vulsellum f.
    Michel clip-applying f.
    Michel clip-removing f.
    Michel tissue f.
    Michigan University
      intestinal f.
    Micrins f.
    micro-Allis f.
    micro-Colibri f.
    micro-Halstead arterial f.
    micro-jewelers monopolar
      f.

forceps (*continued*)
    Micro-Line arterial f.
    Micro-One dissecting f.
    Micro-Two f.
    microarterial f.
    microbayonet f.
    microbiopsy f.
    microbipolar f.
    microbronchoscopic
      grasping f.
    microbronchoscopic tissue
      f.
    microclamp f.
    microclip f.
    microcorneal f.
    microcup pituitary f.
    microdissecting f.
    microdressing f.
    microextractor f.
    microlaryngeal grasping f.
    microneedle holder f.
    microneurosurgical f.
    micropin f.
    Microsnap hemostatic f.
    microsurgical biopsy f.
    microsurgical grasping f.
    microsurgical tying f.
    Microtek cupped f.
    microtip bipolar jeweler's f.
    microtissue f.
    microtying f.
    microvascular clamp-
      applying f.
    microvascular tying f.
    Microvasive disposable
      alligator-shaped f.
    Microvasive radial jaw
      biopsy f.
    midcavity f.
    middle ear strut f.
    Mighty Bite Zimmon lateral
      biopsy cup f.
    Mikulicz peritoneal f.
    Mikulicz tonsillar f.
    Miles punch biopsy f.
    Milex f.
    Mill-Rose RiteBite biopsy f.
    Mill-Rose Surebrite biopsy f.

forceps (*continued*)

Miller articulating f.
Miller bayonet f.
Miller rectal f.
Millin capsular f.
Millin ligature-guiding f.
Millin prostatectomy f.
Millin T-shaped f.
Mills tissue f.
miniature intestinal f.
Mitchell-Diamond biopsy f.
mitral valve-holding f.
Mixter arterial f.
Mixter baby hemostatic f.
Mixter gallbladder f.
Mixter gallstone f.
Mixter mosquito f.
Mixter pediatric hemostatic f.
Mixter thoracic f.
Mixter-McQuigg f.
Mixter-O'Shaughnessy dissecting f.
Mixter-O'Shaughnessy hemostatic f.
Mixter-O'Shaughnessy ligature f.
Mixter-Paul arterial f.
Mixter-Paul hemostatic f.
Moberg f.
Moberg-Stille f.
modified Younge f.
Moehle corneal f.
Moersch bronchoscopic f.
Molt pedicle f.
Monod punch f.
monopolar coagulating f.
monopolar insulated f.
monopolar tissue f.
Montenovesi cranial f.
Moody fixation f.
Moolgaoker f.
Moore lens-inserting f.
Morgenstein blunt f.
Moritz-Schmidt laryngeal f.
Morris f.
Morson f.
Mosher ethmoid punch f.

forceps (*continued*)

mosquito hemostatic f.
Mount intervertebral disk f.
Mount-Mayfield aneurysm f.
Mount-Olivecrona f.
mouse-tooth f.
Moynihan intestinal f.
Moynihan kidney pedicle f.
Moynihan towel f.
Moynihan-Navratil f.
MPC coagulation f.
Muck tonsillar f.
mucous f.
Mueller f.
Mueller-Markham patent ductus f.
Muir hemorrhoidal f.
Muldoon meibomian f.
Multibite multiple sample biopsy f.
multipurpose f.
multitoothed cartilage f.
Mundie placental f.
Murless head extractor f.
Murphy tonsillar f.
Murphy-Péan hemostatic f.
Murray f.
muscle f.
Museholdt nasal-dressing f.
Museux tenaculum f.
Museux uterine f.
Museux vulsellum f.
Museux-Collins uterine vulsellum f.
Musial tissue f.
Mustarde f.
Myerson bronchial f.
Myerson laryngeal f.
Myles hemorrhoidal f.
Myles nasal f.
Nadler bipolar coaptation f.
Naegele obstetrical f.
nail-cutting f.
nail-extracting f.
nail-pulling f.
Nakao Ejector biopsy f.
nasal alligator f.
nasal bone f.

forceps (*continued*)

nasal cartilage-holding f.
nasal hump-cutting f.
nasal insertion f.
nasal lower lateral f.
nasal needle holder f.
nasal polyp f.
nasal septal f.
nasal-cutting f.
nasal-dressing f.
nasal-packing f.
nasopharyngeal biopsy f.
Natvig wire-twister f.
needle f.
needle-holder f.
Negus tonsillar f.
Negus-Green f.
Nelson lung f.
Nelson tissue f.
Nelson-Martin f.
neonatal vascular f.
nephrolithotomy f.
Neubauer foreign body f.
Neubauer vitreous micro-
  extractor f.
Neubuser tube-seizing f.
neurosurgical dressing f.
neurosurgical ligature f.
neurosurgical suction f.
neurosurgical tissue f.
neurovascular f.
Neuwirth-Palmer f.
Neville-Barnes f.
Nevins dressing f.
Nevins tissue f.
Nevyas lens f.
New biopsy f.
New Orleans Eye Ear
  fixation f.
New tissue f.
New York Eye and Ear
  Hospital fixation f.
Newman uterine
  tenaculum f.
Nicola f.
Niedner dissecting f.
NIH mitral valve f.
Niro bone-cutting f.

forceps (*continued*)

Niro wire-twister f.
Niro wire-twisting f.
Nisbet eye f.
Nisbet fixation f.
Nissen cystic f.
Nissen gall duct f.
Nissen hassux f.
Noble iris f.
noncrushing common duct
  f.
noncrushing intestinal f.
noncrushing pickup f.
noncrushing tissue-holding
  f.
nonfenestrated f.
nonmagnetic dressing f.
nonmagnetic tissue f.
nonperforating towel f.
nonslipping f.
nontoothed f.
nontraumatizing visceral f.
Nordan tying f.
Nordan-Colibri f.
Norris sponge f.
Norwood f.
Noto dressing f.
Noto ovum f.
Noto polypus f.
Noto sponge f.
Novak fixation f.
Noyes ear f.
Noyes nasal f.
Noyes nasal-dressing f.
Nugent fixation f.
Nugent rectus f.
Nugent superior rectus f.
Nugent utility f.
Nugowski f.
Nussbaum intestinal f.
Nyhus-Potts intestinal f.
Nystroem tumor f.
Oberhill obstetrical f.
O'Brien fixation f.
O'Brien tissue f.
O'Brien-Elschnig f.
obstetrical f.
occluding f.

forceps (*continued*)

Ochsner arterial f.
Ochsner cartilage f.
Ochsner hemostatic f.
Ochsner tissue f.
Ochsner tissue/cartilage f.
Ochsner-Dixon arterial f.
Ockerblad f.
O'Connor biopsy f.
O'Connor eye f.
O'Connor grasping f.
O'Connor iris f.
O'Connor lid f.
O'Connor sponge f.
O'Connor-Elschnig fixation f.
O'Dell spicule f.
odontoid peg-grasping f.
O'Gawa suture f.
O'Gawa suture-fixation f.
O'Gawa tying f.
O'Gawa-Castroviejo tying f.
Ogura cartilage f.
Ogura tissue f.
O'Hanlon f.
O'Hara f.
Oldberg intervertebral disk f.
Oldberg pituitary rongeur f.
Olivecrona aneurysm f.
Olivecrona clip-applying and removing f.
Olivecrona rongeur f.
Olivecrona-Toennis clip-applying f.
Olsen bayonet monopolar f.
Olympus alligator-jaw endoscopic f.
Olympus basket-type endoscopic f.
Olympus Endo-Therapy disposable biopsy f.
Olympus FB-series biopsy f.
Olympus FG-series f.
Olympus FS-K-series endoscopic suture-cutting f.
Olympus FS-series endoscopic suture-cutting f.

forceps (*continued*)

Olympus grasping rat-tooth f.
Olympus hot biopsy f.
Olympus magnetic extractor f.
Olympus pelican-type endoscopic f.
Olympus rat-tooth endoscopic f.
Olympus reusable oval cup f.
Olympus shark-tooth endoscopic f.
Olympus tripod-type endoscopic f.
Olympus W-shaped endoscopic f.
Ombrédanne f.
optical biopsy f.
oral f.
Orr gall duct f.
orthopedic f.
O'Shaughnessy arterial f.
Osher bipolar coaptation f.
Osher capsular f.
Osher conjunctival f.
Osher foreign body f.
Osher haptic f.
Osher superior rectus f.
ossicle-holding f.
Ossoff-Karlan laser f.
ostrum punch f.
otologic cup f.
Otto tissue f.
Oughterson f.
outlet f.
oval cup f.
ovary f.
Overholt clip-applying f.
Overholt dissecting f.
Overholt-Geissendörfer arterial f.
Overholt-Mixter dissecting f.
Overstreet polyp f.
ovum f.
Pace-Potts f.
Packer mosquito f.

forceps (*continued*)

packing f.
Page tonsillar f.
Palmer biopsy f.
Palmer cutting f.
Palmer grasping f.
Palmer ovarian biopsy f.
Palmer-Drapier f.
Pang biopsy f.
Pang nasopharyngeal f.
Panje-Shagets
   tracheoesophageal fistula
   f.
papilloma f.
parametrium f.
Park lens implantation f.
Parker fixation f.
Parker-Kerr f.
partial-occlusion f.
Passarelli one-pass
   capsulorrhexis f.
passing f.
patent ductus f.
Paterson brain clip f.
Paterson laryngeal f.
Paton anterior chamber
   lens implant f.
Paton capsular f.
Paton corneal f.
Paton corneal transplant f.
Paton extra-delicate f.
Paton suturing f.
Paton tying/stitch removal f.
Patterson bronchoscopic f.
Patterson specimen f.
Paufique suturing f.
Paulson infertility
   microtissue f.
Paulson infertility
   microtying f.
Pauwels fracture f.
Pavlo-Colibri corneal f.
Payne-Ochsner arterial f.
Payne-Pééan arterial f.
Payne-Rankin arterial f.
Payr pylorus f.
Péan arterial f.
Péan hemostatic f.

forceps (*continued*)

Péan hysterectomy f.
Péan intestinal f.
Péan sponge f.
peanut sponge-holding f.
peanut-fenestrated f.
peanut-grasping f.
peapod bead-type f.
peapod intervertebral disk
   f.
pediatric f.
pedicle f.
Peet mosquito f.
Peet splinter f.
pelican biopsy f.
Pelkmann foreign body f.
Pelkmann gallstone f.
Pelkmann sponge f.
Pelkmann uterine f.
pelvic reduction f.
pelvic tissue f.
Pemberton f.
Penfield watchmaker
   suture f.
Penn-Anderson scleral
   fixation f.
Pennington hemorrhoidal f.
Pennington hemostatic f.
Pennington tissue f.
Pennington tissue-grasping
   f.
Percy intestinal f.
Percy tissue f.
Percy-Wolfson gallbladder
   f.
Perdue tonsillar hemostat f.
Perez-Castro f.
peripheral blood vessel f.
peripheral iridectomy f.
peripheral vascular f.
peritoneal f.
Perman cartilage f.
Perone LASIK flap f.
Perritt fixation f.
Perritt lens f.
Perry f.
Peter-Bishop f.
Peters tissue f.

forceps (*continued*)
Peyman intraocular f.
Peyman vitreous-grasping f.
Peyman-Green vitreous f.
Pfau polyp f.
Pfister-Schwartz basket f.
phalangeal f.
Phaneuf arterial f.
Phaneuf hysterectomy f.
Phaneuf peritoneal f.
Phaneuf uterine artery f.
Phaneuf vaginal f.
Phillips fixation f.
Phillips swan neck f.
phimosis f.
Phipps f.
phrenicectomy f.
pickup noncrushing f.
Pierse corneal Colibri-type f.
Pierse fixation f.
Pierse tip f.
Pierse-Colibri corneal utility f.
Pierse-Hoskins f.
Pigott f.
Pike jawed f.
pillar f.
pillar-grasping f.
Pilling f.
Pilling-Liston bone utility f.
pin-bending f.
pin-seating f.
pinch f.
Piper obstetrical f.
Piranha uteroscopic biopsy f.
Pischel micropin f.
Pistofidis cervical biopsy f.
Pitanguy f.
Pitha foreign body f.
Pitha urethral f.
pituitary f.
placement f.
placenta previa f.
plain f.
plastic f.
plate-holding f.

forceps (*continued*)
platform f.
pleurectomy f.
Pley capsular f.
Pley extracapsular f.
Plondke uterine f.
point f.
Polaris reusable f.
Polk placental f.
Polk sponge f.
Pollock double corneal f.
polyp f.
polypus f.
Poppen intervertebral disk f.
Porter duodenal f.
Post f.
posterior f.
postnasal sponge f.
Potta coarctation f.
Potter sponge f.
Potter tonsillar f.
Potts bronchial f.
Potts bulldog f.
Potts coarctation f.
Potts fixation f.
Potts intestinal f.
Potts patent ductus f.
Potts thumb f.
Potts-Nevins dressing f.
Potts-Smith bipolar f.
Potts-Smith dressing f.
Potts-Smith monopolar f.
Potts-Smith tissue f.
Poutasse renal artery f.
Pozzi tenaculum f.
Pratt hemostatic f.
Pratt T-shaped hemostatic f.
Pratt tissue f.
Pratt vulsellum f.
Pratt-Smith hemostatic f.
Precisor Direct Bite biopsy f.
Prentiss f.
prepuce f.
Presbyterian Hospital f.
pressure f.
Preston ligamentum flavum f.

forceps (*continued*)

Price-Thomas bronchial f.
Primbs suturing f.
Prince advancement f.
Prince muscle f.
Prince trachoma f.
proctological grasping f.
proctological polyp f.
Proctor phrenectomy f.
Proctor phrenicectomy f.
prostatectomy f.
prostatic lobe f.
protological biopsy f.
Proud adenoidectomy f.
Providence Hospital arterial f.
ptosis f.
pulmonary arterial f.
pulmonary vessel f.
punch f.
Puntenney tying f.
Puntowicz arterial f.
pupil spreader/retractor f.
QSA dressing f.
quadripolar cutting f.
Quervain cranial f.
Quevedo conjunctival f.
Quevedo fixation f.
Quevedo suturing f.
Quinones uterine-grasping f.
Quinones-Neubüser uterine-grasping f.
Quire foreign body f.
Quire mechanical finger f.
Raaf f.
Raaf-Oldberg intervertebral disk f.
Radial Jaw bladder biopsy f.
Radial Jaw hot biopsy f.
Radial Jaw single-use biopsy f.
Raimondi scalp hemostatic f.
Ralks ear f.
Ralks splinter f.
Ralks wire-cutting f.
Rampley sponge f.

forceps (*continued*)

Rand f.
Randall stone f.
Raney rongeur f.
Raney scalp clip-applying f.
Raney straight coagulating f.
Rankin arterial f.
Rankin hemostatic f.
Rankin-Crile f.
Rankow f.
Rapp f.
Rappazzo intraocular foreign body f.
rat-tooth f.
Ratliff-Blake gallstone f.
Ratliff-Mayo gallstone f.
Ray kidney stone f.
reach-and-pin f.
Read f.
recession f.
rectal f.
Reese advancement f.
Reese muscle f.
Reich-Nechtow hypogastric artery f.
Reich-Nechtow hysterectomy f.
Reill f.
Reiner-Knight ethmoid-cutting f.
Reinhoff arterial f.
Reisinger lens-extracting f.
renal artery f.
Resano sigmoid f.
resection intestinal f.
retrieval f.
Reul coronary f.
reverse-action hypophysectomy f.
Rezek f.
Rhein capsulorhexis cystitome f.
Rhein fine foldable lens-insertion f.
Rhoton bipolar f.
Rhoton cup f.
Rhoton dural f.

forceps (*continued*)

Rhoton grasping f.
Rhoton microcup f.
Rhoton microdissecting f.
Rhoton microtying f.
Rhoton microvascular f.
Rhoton ring tumor f.
Rhoton tissue f.
Rhoton transsphenoidal bipolar f.
Rhoton tying f.
Rhoton-Adson dressing f.
Rhoton-Adson tissue f.
Rhoton-Cushing tissue f.
Rhoton-Tew bipolar f.
rib rongeur f.
Riba-Valeira f.
Rica clip-applying f.
Rica hemostatic f.
Rica-Adson f.
Rich f.
Richards f.
Richards tonsillar f.
Richards-Andrews f.
Riches artery f.
Riches diathermy f.
Richmond f.
Richter f.
Richter-Heath clip-removing f.
ridge f.
Ridley f.
right-angle f.
rigid biopsy f.
rigid kidney stone f.
ring f.
ring-rotation f.
ring-tip f.
ringed formed f.
Ringenberg stapedectomy f.
Ripstein arterial f.
Ripstein tissue f.
Ritch-Krupin-Denver eye valve insertion f.
RiteBite biopsy f.
Ritter f.
Rizzuti double-prong f.
Rizzuti fixation f.

forceps (*continued*)

Rizzuti scleral f.
Rizzuti superior rectus f.
Rizzuti-Furness cornea-holding f.
Rizzuti-Verhoeff f.
Robb tonsillar f.
Roberts arterial f.
Roberts bronchial f.
Roberts hemostatic f.
Roberts-Singley dressing f.
Roberts-Singley thumb f.
Robertson tonsillar f.
Robson intestinal f.
Rochester gallstone f.
Rochester oral tissue f.
Rochester Russian tissue f.
Rochester tissue f.
Rochester-Carmalt hysterectomy f.
Rochester-Davis f.
Rochester-Ewald tissue f.
Rochester-Harrington f.
Rochester-Mixter arterial f.
Rochester-Mixter gall duct f.
Rochester-Mueller f.
Rochester-Ochsner f.
Rochester-Péan hysterectomy f.
Rochester-Rankin arterial f.
Rockey f.
Roeder f.
Roeltsch f.
Roger vascular-toothed hysterectomy f.
Rolf jeweler's f.
Rolf utility f.
roller f.
rongeur f.
Ronis cutting f.
Rose disimpaction f.
rotating f.
Roubaix f.
round punch f.
round-handled f.
Rovenstine catheter-introducing f.
Rowe bone-drilling f.

forceps (*continued*)
    Rowe disimpaction f.
    Rowe glenoid-reaming f.
    Rowe maxillary f.
    Rowe modified-Harrison f.
    Rowe-Harrison bone-
        holding f.
    Rowe-Killey f.
    Rowland double-action f.
    Rowland hump f.
    Royce f.
    rubber-shod f.
    Rudd Clinic hemorrhoidal f.
    Ruel f.
    Rugby deep-surgery f.
    Rugelski arterial f.
    Rumel dissecting f.
    Rumel lobectomy f.
    Rumel thoracic f.
    Ruskin bone-cutting f.
    Ruskin rongeur f.
    Ruskin-Liston bone-cutting
        f.
    Ruskin-Rowland bone-
        cutting f.
    Russ tumor f.
    Russ vascular f.
    Russell f.
    Russell hysterectomy f.
    Russell-Davis f.
    Russian Péan f.
    Russian thumb f.
    Russian tissue f.
    Rycroft tying f.
    ST Lalonde hook f.
    Sachs tissue f.
    Saenger ovum f.
    Saenger placental f.
    Sajou laryngeal f.
    Sam Roberts bronchial
        biopsy f.
    Samuels hemoclip-applying
        f.
    Sanders vasectomy f.
    Sanders-Castroviejo
        suturing f.
    Sandt suture f.
    Sandt utility f.

forceps (*continued*)
    Santy ring-end f.
    Saqalain dressing f.
    Sarot arterial f.
    Sarot intrathoracic f.
    Sarot pleurectomy f.
    Satellight needle holder f.
    Satinsky f.
    Satterlee advancement f.
    Satterlee muscle f.
    Sauer outer ring f.
    Sauer suture f.
    Sauer suturing f.
    Sauerbruch pickup f.
    Sauerbruch rib f.
    Sawtell arterial f.
    Sawtell gallbladder f.
    Sawtell tonsillar f.
    Sawtell-Davis f.
    scalp clip-applying f.
    Scanlan laparoscopic f.
    Scanzoni f.
    Schaaf foreign body f.
    Schaefer fixation f.
    Schanzioni craniotomy f.
    Scharff bipolar f.
    Schatz utility f.
    Scheer crimper f.
    Scheie-Graefe fixation f.
    Scheinmann
        esophagoscopy f.
    Scheinmann laryngeal f.
    Schepens f.
    Schick f.
    Schindler peritoneal f.
    Schlesinger cervical punch
        f.
    Schlesinger intervertebral
        disk f.
    Schlesinger meniscus-
        grasping f.
    Schlesinger rongeur f.
    Schnidt gall duct f.
    Schnidt thoracic f.
    Schnidt tonsillar f.
    Schnidt-Rumpler f.
    Schoenberg intestinal f.
    Schoenberg uterine f.

forceps (*continued*)

Scholten endomyocardial biopsy f.
Schroeder tissue f.
Schroeder uterine vulsellum f.
Schroeder-Braun uterine f.
Schroeder-Van Doren tenaculum f.
Schubert cervical biopsy f.
Schubert uterine biopsy f.
Schumacher biopsy f.
Schutz f.
Schwartz clip-applying f.
Schwartz multipurpose f.
Schwartz obstetrical f.
Schwartz temporary clamp-applying f.
Schweigger capsule f.
Schweigger extracapsular f.
Schweizer cervix-holding f.
Schweizer uterine f.
scissors f.
scleral twist-grip f.
sclerectomy punch f.
Scobee-Allis f.
Scott lens-insertion f.
Scoville brain f.
Scoville clip-applying f.
Scoville-Greenwood bayonet neurosurgical bipolar f.
Scoville-Hurteau f.
screw-holding f.
Scudder intestinal f.
Scuderi bipolar coagulating f.
Searcy capsular f.
Segond hysterectomy f.
Segond tumor f.
Segond-Landau hysterectomy f.
Seiffert esophagoscopy f.
Seiffert laryngeal f.
Seitzinger tripolar cutting f.
seizing f.
Seletz foramen-plugging f.
self-opening f.

forceps (*continued*)

self-retaining bone f.
Selman nonslip tissue f.
Selman peripheral blood vessel f.
Selman tissue f.
Selman vessel f.
Selverstone embolus f.
Selverstone intervertebral disk f.
Selverstone rongeur f.
Semb bone f.
Semb bone-cutting f.
Semb bone-holding f.
Semb dissecting f.
Semb ligature f.
Semb ligature-carrying f.
Semb rib f.
Semb rongeur f.
Semb-Ghazi dissecting f.
Semken bipolar f.
Semken dressing f.
Semken infant f.
Semken microbipolar neurosurgical f.
Semken thumb f.
Semken tissue f.
Semmes dural f.
Senning cardiovascular f.
Senturia f.
septal bone f.
septal compression f.
septal ridge f.
septum-cutting f.
septum-straightening f.
sequestrum f.
serrated conjunctival f.
serrefine f.
Sewall brain clip-applying f.
Seyfert f.
Shaaf eye f.
Shaaf foreign body f.
Shallcross cystic duct f.
Shallcross gallbladder f.
Shallcross nasal f.
Shallcross-Dean gall duct f.
Shapshay-Healy laryngeal alligator f.

forceps (*continued*)

    Shark f.
    shark-tooth f.
    sharp-pointed f.
    Shearer chicken-bill f.
    Sheehy ossicle-holding f.
    Sheets lens f.
    Sheets-McPherson angled f.
    Sheets-McPherson tying f.
    Sheinmann laryngeal f.
    Shepard bipolar f.
    Shepard curved intraocular
      lens f.
    Shepard lens f.
    Shepard tying f.
    Shepard-Reinstein
      intraocular lens f.
    Shields f.
    Shoemaker intraocular lens
      f.
    short tooth f.
    Shuppe biting f.
    Shuster suture f.
    Shuster tonsillar f.
    Shutt Aggressor f.
    Shutt alligator f.
    Shutt B-scoop f.
    Shutt basket f.
    Shutt grasping f.
    Shutt Mantis retrograde f.
    Shutt Mini-Aggressor f.
    Shutt retrograde f.
    Shutt shovel-nosed f.
    Shutt suction f.
    side-biting Stammberger
      punch f.
    side-curved f.
    side-cutting basket f.
    side-grasping f.
    side-lip f.
    Siegler biopsy f.
    Silcock dissection f.
    silicone rod and sleeve f.
    silicone sponge f.
    Silver endaural f.
    Simcoe implantation f.
    Simcoe lens-inserting f.
    Simcoe nucleus f.

forceps (*continued*)

    Simcoe posterior chamber
      f.
    Simcoe superior rectus f.
    Simons stone-removing f.
    Simpson obstetrical f.
    Simpson-Braun obstetrical
      f.
    Simpson-Luikart obstetrical
      f.
    Sims-Maier sponge and
      dressing f.
    single-tooth f.
    Singley intestinal f.
    Singley tissue f.
    Singley-Tuttle dressing f.
    Singley-Tuttle intestinal f.
    Singley-Tuttle tissue f.
    Sinskey intraocular lens f.
    Sinskey microtying f.
    Sinskey-McPherson f.
    Sinskey-Wilson foreign
      body f.
    sinus biopsy f.
    Sisson f.
    sister-hook f.
    Skeleton fine f.
    Skene tenaculum f.
    Skene uterine f.
    Skene vulsellum f.
    Skillern phimosis f.
    Skillman arterial f.
    Skillman mosquito f.
    Skillman prepuce f.
    skin f.
    sleeve-spreading f.
    sliding capsular f.
    Sluder-Ballenger tonsillar
      punch f.
    small cup biopsy f.
    Smart chalazion f.
    Smart nonslipping
      chalazion f.
    Smellie obstetrical f.
    Smith Nephew Richards
      bipolar f.
    Smith grasping f.
    Smith lion-jaw f.

forceps (*continued*)

Smith obstetrical f.
Smith-Leiske cross-action
  intraocular lens f.
Smith-Petersen f.
Smithwick clip-applying f.
Smithwick-Hartmann f.
smooth dressing f.
smooth tissue f.
smooth-tipped jeweler's f.
smooth-tooth f.
Snellen entropion f.
Snyder corneal spring f.
Snyder deep-surgery f.
Somers uterine f.
Songer tonsillar f.
Soonawalla vasectomy f.
Sopher ovum f.
Sourdille f.
Spaleck f.
Sparta micro-iris f.
spatula f.
specimen f.
speculum f.
Spence rongeur f.
Spence-Adson f.
Spencer biopsy f.
Spencer chalazion f.
Spencer plication f.
Spencer-Wells arterial f.
Spencer-Wells chalazion f.
Spero meibomian f.
Spetzler f.
sphenoidal punch f.
spicule f.
spinal-perforating f.
spiral f.
splaytooth f.
splinter f.
splitting f.
sponge f.
sponge-holding f.
spoon f.
spoon-shaped f.
spreading f.
spring-handled f.
Spurling intervertebral disk
  f.

forceps (*continued*)

Spurling rongeur f.
Spurling tissue f.
Spurling-Kerrison rongeur f.
square specimen f.
squeeze-handle f.
St. Clair f.
St. Clair-Thompson
  adenoidal f.
St. Clair-Thompson
  peritonsillar abscess f.
St. Martin eye f.
St. Martin suturing f.
St. Vincent tube-occluding
  f.
Stamm bone-cutting f.
Stammberger side-biting
  punch f.
standard arterial f.
stapedectomy f.
stapes f.
staple f.
Stark vulsellum f.
Starr fixation f.
Staude tenaculum f.
Staude-Jackson tenaculum
  f.
Staude-Moore uterine
  tenaculum f.
Stavis fixation f.
Steinmann intestinal f.
Steinmann tendon f.
Stephens soft IOL-inserting
  f.
sterilizing f.
Stern-Castroviejo locking f.
Stern-Castroviejo suturing f.
sternal punch f.
Stevens fixation f.
Stevens iris f.
Stevenson alligator f.
Stevenson cupped-jaw f.
Stevenson grasping f.
Stevenson microsurgical f.
Stieglitz splinter f.
Stille gallstone f.
Stille kidney f.
Stille rongeur f.

forceps (*continued*)

Stille tissue f.
Stille-Adson f.
Stille-Babcock f.
Stille-Barraya intestinal f.
Stille-Barraya vascular f.
Stille-Björk f.
Stille-Crafoord f.
Stille-Crile f.
Stille-Halsted f.
Stille-Horsley bone-cutting f.
Stille-Horsley rib f.
Stille-Liston bone f.
Stille-Liston rib-cutting f.
Stille-Luer rongeur f.
Stille-Russian f.
Stille-Waugh f.
Stiwer biopsy f.
Stiwer bone-holding f.
Stiwer dressing f.
Stiwer sponge f.
Stiwer tissue f.
Stolte capsulorhexis f.
Stone clamp-applying f.
Stone intestinal f.
Stone tissue f.
stone-crushing f.
stone-extraction f.
stone-grasping f.
Stoneman f.
Storey gall duct f.
Storey thoracic f.
Storey-Hillar dissecting f.
Storz biopsy f.
Storz bronchoscopic f.
Storz capsular f.
Storz ciliary f.
Storz corneal f.
Storz curved f.
Storz cystoscopic f.
Storz esophagoscopic f.
Storz grasping biopsy f.
Storz kidney stone f.
Storz Microsystems plate-holding f.
Storz miniature f.
Storz nasopharyngeal biopsy f.

forceps (*continued*)

Storz optical biopsy f.
Storz sinus biopsy f.
Storz stone-crushing f.
Storz stone-extraction f.
Storz-Bonn suturing f.
Storz-Utrata f.
strabismus f.
straight coagulating f.
straight knot-tying f.
straight line bayonet f.
straight Maryland f.
straight microbipolar f.
straight micromonopolar f.
straight single tenaculum f.
straight tying f.
straight-end cup f.
straight-tip bipolar f.
straight-tip jeweler's bipolar f.
Strassburger tissue f.
Strassmann uterine f.
Stratte f.
Streli f.
Strelinger catheter-introducing f.
Stringer catheter-introducing f.
Stringer newborn throat f.
Strow corneal f.
Struempel ear alligator f.
Struempel ear punch f.
Struempel-Voss ethmoidal f.
Struempel-Voss nasal f.
Strully dressing f.
Strully tissue f.
strut f.
Struyken ear f.
Struyken nasal f.
Struyken nasal-cutting f.
Struyken turbinate f.
Styles f.
subglottic f.
suction f.
Suker iris f.
superior rectus f.
SureBite biopsy f.

forceps (*continued*)

    Sutherland vitreous f.
    Sutherland-Grieshaber f.
    suture clip f.
    suture tag f.
    suture-tying platform f.
    suturing f.
    Swan-Brown arterial f.
    Sweet clip-applying f.
    Sweet dissecting f.
    Sweet ligature f.
    Syark vulsellum f.
    synovium biopsy f.
    Szuler vascular f.
    Szultz corneal f.
    T-shaped f.
    tack-and-pin f.
    Takahashi cutting f.
    Takahashi ethmoidal f.
    Takahashi iris retractor f.
    Takahashi nasal f.
    Takahashi neurosurgical f.
    Take-apart f.
    tampon f.
    Tamsco f.
    tangential f.
    taper-jaw f.
    Tarnier axis-traction f.
    Tarnier obstetrical f.
    Taylor dissecting f.
    Taylor tissue f.
    Taylor-Cushing dressing f.
    Teale tenaculum f.
    Teale uterine f.
    Teale vulsellum f.
    Tekno f.
    tenaculum f.
    tenaculum-reducing f.
    tendon f.
    tendon-holding f.
    tendon-passing f.
    tendon-pulling f.
    tendon-retrieving f.
    tendon-seizing f.
    Tennant intraocular lens f.
    Tennant lens f.
    Tennant titanium suturing f.
    Tennant tying f.

forceps (*continued*)

    Tennant-Colibri corneal f.
    Tennant-Maumenee f.
    Tennant-Troutman superior rectus f.
    Tenzel bipolar f.
    Terson capsular f.
    Terson extracapsular f.
    Thackray dental f.
    The Shark disposable biopsy f.
    Therma Jaw hot urologic f.
    Theurig sterilizer f.
    Thomas fixation f.
    Thomas shot compression f.
    Thompson hip prosthesis f.
    Thoms tissue f.
    Thoms-Allis intestinal f.
    Thoms-Allis tissue f.
    Thoms-Gaylor uterine f.
    thoracic artery f.
    thoracic tissue f.
    Thorek gallbladder f.
    Thorek-Mixter gallbladder f.
    Thornton episcleral f.
    Thornton fixation f.
    Thornton intraocular f.
    Thorpe conjunctival f.
    Thorpe corneal f.
    Thorpe corneoscleral f.
    Thorpe foreign body f.
    Thorpe-Castroviejo corneal f.
    Thorpe-Castroviejo fixation f.
    Thorpe-Castroviejo vitreous foreign body f.
    Thrasher intraocular f.
    Thrasher lens implant f.
    three-prong grasping f.
    throat f.
    thumb tissue f.
    Thurston-Holland fragment f.
    thyroid f.
    Tickner tissue f.
    Tiemann bullet f.

forceps (*continued*)
  Tiger Shark f.
  Tilley dressing f.
  Tilley-Henckel f.
  Tischler cervical biopsy
     punch f.
  Tischler-Morgan uterine
     biopsy f.
  tissue f.
  tissue-grasping f.
  tissue-holding f.
  tissue-spreading f.
  titanium microsurgical
     bipolar f.
  Tivnen tonsillar f.
  Tobey ear f.
  Tobold laryngeal f.
  Tobold-Fauvel grasping f.
  Toennis tumor-grasping f.
  Toennis-Adson f.
  Tomac f.
  tongue f.
  tonsil f.
  tonsillar abscess f.
  tonsillar artery f.
  tonsillar hemostatic f.
  tonsillar pillar grasping f.
  tonsillar punch f.
  Tooke corneal f.
  Toomey f.
  tooth-extracting f.
  toothed thumb f.
  toothed tissue f.
  toothless f.
  Torchia capsular f.
  Torchia lens implantation f.
  Torchia microbipolar f.
  Torchia tissue f.
  Torchia tying f.
  Torchia-Colibri f.
  Torres cross-action f.
  torsion f.
  Tower muscle f.
  Townley tissue f.
  tracheal f.
  trachoma f.
  traction f.
  transfer f.

forceps (*continued*)
  transsphenoidal bipolar f.
  traumatic grasping f.
  triangular punch f.
  tripod grasping f.
  Troeltsch dressing f.
  Troeltsch ear f.
  Trotter f.
  Trousseau dilating f.
  Troutman corneal f.
  Troutman microsurgery f.
  Troutman superior rectus f.
  Troutman tying f.
  Troutman-Barraquer
     corneal fixation f.
  Troutman-Barraquer
     corneal f.
  Troutman-Barraquer iris f.
  Troutman-Barraquer-Colibri
     f.
  Troutman-Llobera fixation f.
  Troutman-Llobera-Flieringa
     f.
  Truline f.
  Trush grasping f.
  Trylon hemostatic f.
  tube-occluding f.
  tubing f.
  tubing introducer f.
  Tubinger gall stone f.
  tubular f.
  Tucker bead f.
  Tucker hallux f.
  Tucker reach-and-pin f.
  Tucker staple f.
  Tucker tack and pin f.
  Tucker-McLane axis-
     traction f.
  Tucker-McLane obstetrical
     f.
  Tucker-McLane-Luikart f.
  Tudor-Edwards bone-
     cutting f.
  Tuffier arterial f.
  tumor f.
  tumor-grasping f.
  turbinate f.
  Turnbull adhesion f.

forceps (*continued*)

Turner-Babcock tissue f.
Turner-Warwick stone f.
Turner-Warwick-Adson f.
Turrell rectal biopsy f.
Turrell specimen f.
Turrell-Wittner rectal biopsy f.
Tuttle dressing f.
Tuttle obstetrical f.
Tuttle thoracic f.
Tuttle thumb f.
Tuttle tissue f.
Tuttle-Singley thoracic f.
Twisk f.
two-stream irrigating f.
two-toothed f.
Tydings tonsillar f.
Tydings-Lakeside tonsillar f.
tying f.
tympanoplasty f.
Tyrrell foreign body f.
U-shaped f.
Ullrich dressing f.
Ullrich-Aesculap f.
Ullrich-St. Gallen f.
Ulrich bone-holding f.
Ultrata capsulorhexis f.
Universal f.
University of Kansas corneal f.
University of Michigan Mixter thoracic f.
up-cupped f.
upbiting biopsy f.
upbiting cup f.
upcurved basket f.
Uppsala gall duct f.
upturned f.
upward bent f.
Urbantschitsch nasal f.
ureteral catheter f.
ureteral isolation f.
ureteral stone f.
uterine artery f.
uterine biopsy punch f.
uterine polyp f.
uterine specimen f.

forceps (*continued*)

uterine tenaculum f.
uterine vulsellum f.
uterine-dressing f.
uterine-elevating f.
uterine-grasping f.
uterine-holding f.
uterine-manipulating f.
uterine-packing f.
utility f.
Utrata capsulorhexis f.
vaginal hysterectomy f.
Valin f.
Van Buren bone-holding f.
Van Buren sequestrum f.
Vander Pool sterilizer f.
Vanderbilt arterial f.
Vanderbilt deep-vessel f.
Vanderbilt University hemostatic f.
Vanderbilt University vessel f.
Van Doren uterine biopsy punch f.
Vannas fixation f.
Van Ruben f.
Van Struyken nasal f.
Vantage tube-occluding f.
Vantec grasping f.
Varco gallbladder f.
Varco thoracic f.
vascular tissue f.
vasectomy f.
vas isolation f.
Vaughn sterilizer f.
vectis cesarean f.
vena cava f.
Verbrugge bone-holding f.
Verhoeff capsular f.
Verhoeff capsule f.
Verhoeff cataract f.
vertical f.
vessel f.
Vick-Blanchard hemorrhoidal f.
Vickerall round ringed f.
Vickers ring-tip f.
Victor-Bonney f.

forceps (*continued*)
Vigger-5 eye f.
Virtus splinter f.
viscera-holding f.
visceral f.
vise f.
visual hemostatic f.
Vital general tissue f.
Vital intestinal f.
Vital lung-grasping f.
Vital needle holder f.
Vital-Adson tissue f.
Vital-Babcock tissue f.
Vital-Cushing tissue f.
Vital-Duval intestinal f.
Vital-Evans pelvic tissue f.
Vital-Potts-Smith f.
Vital-Wangensteen tissue f.
vitreous-grasping f.
Vogler hysterectomy f.
Vogt toothed capsular f.
vomer septal f.
von Graefe fixation f.
von Graefe iris f.
von Graefe tissue f.
Von Mandach capsule
   fragment f.
Von Mandach clot f.
von Petz f.
Voris-Oldberg intervertebral
   disk f.
Vorse tube-occluding f.
Vorse-Webster f.
VPI-Ambrose resectoscope
   f.
vulsellum f.
W-shape f.
Wachtenfeldt clip-applying
   f.
Wadsworth lid f.
Wainstock eye suturing f.
Waldeau fixation f.
Waldenstrom laryngeal f.
Waldeyer f.
Walker f.
Wallace cesarean f.
Walsh tissue f.
Walsham nasal f.

forceps (*continued*)
Walsham septal f.
Walsham septum-
   straightening f.
Walter splinter f.
Walther tissue f.
Walton meniscal f.
Walton-Allis tissue f.
Walton-Liston f.
Walton-Schubert uterine
   biopsy f.
Walzl hysterectomy f.
Wangensteen intestinal f.
Wangensteen tissue f.
Warthen f.
watchmaker f.
Watson duckbill f.
Watson tonsil-seizing f.
Watson-Williams ethmoid-
   biting f.
Watson-Williams nasal f.
Watson-Williams polyp f.
Watzke f.
Waugh dissection f.
Waugh dressing f.
Waugh tissue f.
Waugh-Brophy f.
wave-tooth f.
Weaver chalazion f.
Weck hysterectomy f.
Weck rectal biopsy f.
Weck towel f.
Weck uterine biopsy f.
Weck-Harms f.
Weeks eye f.
Weiger-Zollner f.
Weil ear f.
Weil ethmoidal f.
Weil-Blakesley ethmoidal f.
Weiner uterine biopsy f.
Weingartner ear f.
Weis chalazion f.
Weisman f.
Weiss f.
Welch Allyn anal biopsy f.
Weller cartilage f.
Weller meniscal f.
Wells f.

forceps (*continued*)
    Welsh ophthalmic f.
    Welsh pupil-spreader f.
    Wertheim hysterectomy f.
    Wertheim uterine f.
    Wertheim vaginal f.
    Wertheim-Cullen
        compression f.
    Wertheim-Cullen
        hysterectomy f.
    Wertheim-Cullen kidney
        pedicle f.
    Wertheim-Navratil f.
    West nasal-dressing f.
    Westermark uterine
        dressing f.
    Westermark-Stille f.
    Westmacott dressing f.
    Westphal gall duct f.
    Westphal hemostatic f.
    Wheeler plaque f.
    Wheeler vessel f.
    White tonsillar f.
    White-Lillie tonsillar f.
    White-Oslay prostatic f.
    White-Smith f.
    Whitney superior rectus f.
    Wickman uterine f.
    Wiener hysterectomy f.
    Wies chalazion f.
    Wiet otologic cup f.
    Wikström arterial f.
    Wilde ear f.
    Wilde ethmoidal
        exenteration f.
    Wilde intervertebral disk f.
    Wilde laminectomy f.
    Wilde nasal-cutting f.
    Wilde nasal-dressing f.
    Wilde septal f.
    Wilde-Blakesley ethmoidal
        f.
    Wilde-Troeltsch f.
    Wilder dilating f.
    Wilkerson intraocular lens-
        insertion f.
    Willauer intrathoracic f.
    Willauer-Allis thoracic f.

forceps (*continued*)
    Willauer-Allis tissue f.
    Willett placenta previa f.
    Willett placental f.
    Willett scalp flap f.
    Williams diskectomy f.
    Williams gastrointestinal f.
    Williams intestinal f.
    Williams splinter f.
    Williams tissue f.
    Williams uterine f.
    Williams vessel-holding f.
    Williamsburg f.
    Wills Hospital ophthalmic f.
    Wills utility f.
    Wilmer iris f.
    Wilson vitreous foreign
        body f.
    Wilson-Cook bronchoscope
        biopsy f.
    Wilson-Cook colonoscope
        biopsy f.
    Wilson-Cook gastroscope
        biopsy f.
    Wilson-Cook grasping f.
    Wilson-Cook hot biopsy f.
    Wilson-Cook retrieval f.
    Wilson-Cook tripod
        retrieval f.
    Winter ovum f.
    Winter placental f.
    Winter-Nassauer placental f.
    wire prosthesis-crimping f.
    wire-closure f.
    wire-crimping f.
    wire-pulling f.
    wire-twisting f.
    Wittner uterine biopsy f.
    Wolf biopsy f.
    Wolf biting-basket f.
    Wolf cataract delivery f.
    Wolf curved-basket f.
    Wolf eye f.
    Wolf uterine cuff f.
    Wolfson f.
    Woodward f.
    Woodward thoracic artery
        f.

forceps (*continued*)
    Woodward-Potts intestinal f.
    Worth advancement f.
    Worth muscle f.
    Worth strabismus f.
    wound f.
    wound-clip f.
    Wright-Rubin f.
    Wrigley f.
    Wullstein ear f.
    Wullstein tympanoplasty f.
    Wullstein-House f.
    Wullstein-Paparella f.
    Wylie tenaculum f.
    Wylie uterine f.
    X-long cement f.
    Yankauer ethmoidal f.
    Yankauer-Little f.
    Yasargil angled f.
    Yasargil applying f.
    Yasargil arterial f.
    Yasargil bipolar f.
    Yasargil clip-applying f.
    Yasargil flat serrated ring f.
    Yasargil microvessel clip-applying f.
    Yasargil neurosurgical bipolar f.
    Yasargil straight f.
    Yeoman uterine biopsy f.
    Yeoman uterine f.
    Yeoman-Wittner rectal f.
    Young intestinal f.

forceps (*continued*)
    Young lobe f.
    Young prostatectomy f.
    Young prostatic f.
    Young tongue f.
    Young uterine f.
    Younge uterine f.
    Younge-Kevorkian f.
    Z-clamp hysterectomy f.
    Zeeifel angiotribe f.
    Zenker f.
    Zeppelin obstetrical f.
    Ziegler ciliary f.
    Zimmer-Hoen f.
    Zimmer-Schlesinger f.
    Zollinger multipurpose tissue

Freeway PTCA Catheter

Freezor cryocatheter

Frostline linear cryoablation system

Fujinon
    F. biopsy forceps
    F. Sonoprobe

Fukushima
    F.-Giannotta curette
    F.-Giannotta dissector
    F.-Giannotta needle holder
    F.-Giannotta scissors

Futura resectoscope sheath

G

GAIT spacer

Galileo rigid hysteroscope

Gallannaugh bone plate

Gardner
- G. bone chisel
- G. chair
- G. headrest
- G. hysterectomy forceps
- G. needle holder
- G. skull clamp

gastroscope
- ACMI g.
- Bernstein g.
- Chevalier Jackson g.
- Eder g.
- Ellsner g.
- Ewald g.
- Fujinon EG-series g.
- Fujinon GF-series g.
- Hirschowitz g.
- Housset-Debray g.
- Janeway g.
- Mancke flex-rigid g.
- Schindler g.
- Sielaff g.
- Taylor g.
- Tomenius g.
- Universal g.
- Wolf-Henning g.
- Wolf-Knittlingen g.
- Wolf-Schindler g.

gauze
- Adaptic g.
- Aquaphor g.
- Avant Gauze nonwoven g.
- Cover-Roll adhesive g.
- GraftCyte g.
- Intersorb fine mesh g.
- Intersorb six-ply absorbent roll g.
- Intersorb wide mesh g.
- Kling g.
- Oxycel g.

gauze (*continued*)
- PanoGauze hydrogel-impregnated g.
- Safe-Wrap g.
- Sof-Form conforming g.
- Sta-tite 2 ply elastic roll g.
- Surgicel g.
- Surgitube tubular g.
- Teletrast g.
- Telfa g.
- Telfa g.
- Topper nonadherent g.
- TransiGel hydrogel-impregnated g.
- White Plume absorbent g.
- Xeroform g.

Gelfilm
- G. cap
- G. dressing
- G. forceps
- G. plate
- G. retinal implant

Gelfoam
- G. cookie
- G. cube
- G. pad
- G. punch
- G. torpedo

Gellhorn
- G. pessary
- G. uterine biopsy forceps
- G. uterine biopsy punch

Gelocast
- G. cast material
- G. Unna boot

Gemini
- G. clamp
- G. DDD pacemaker
- G. hemostatic forceps
- G. Mixter forceps
- G. paired helical wire basket
- G. thoracic forceps

Gensini cardiac device

Georgiade
G. breast prosthesis
G. fixation device
G. rasp
G. visor
G. visor cervical traction
G. visor halo fixation
apparatus

Ghajar guide

Gherini-Kauffman endo-
otoprobe

Gianturco
G. expandable metallic
biliary stent
G. wool-tufted wire coil
G. zigzag stent
G.-Roehm vena cava filter
G.-Roubin flexible coil stent
G. Z-stent

Giebel blade plate

Girard fragmatome

Glassman stone extractor

Godina double hook vessel-
fixation system

Goetz cardiac device

Goodale-Lubin cardiac device

Gore Smoother Crucial Tool

Gore-Tex
G. bifurcated vascular graft
G. cardiovascular patch
G. catheter
G. DualMesh Plus
G. FEP-Ringed vascular
graft
G. knee prosthesis
G. limb
G. MycroMesh Plus
G. nasal implant
G. SAM facial implant
G. shunt
G. soft tissue patch

Gore-Tex (*continued*)
G. stretch vascular graft
G. strip
G. surgical membrane
G. tapered vascular graft

Gottschalk Nasostat

Gott shunt

Graefe
G. cataract knife
G. cystitome knife
G. eye speculum
G. iris hook
G. scarifier
G. strabismus hook
G. straight iris forceps
G. tissue forceps

graft
AlloDerm processed tissue
g.
AlloMatrix injectable putty
bone graft substitute
Apligraf
Aria g.
atrium (wrapped) Advanta
g.
autologous fat g.
Bard Composix mesh g.
Bard Sperma-Tex
preshaped mesh g.
Bard Visilex mesh g.
Biobrane g.
Biograft bovine heterograft
BioPolyMeric g.
BonePlast g.
Bonfiglio g.
Calcitite
Carbo-Seal cardiovascular
composite g.
Cardiopass g.
Collagraft bone graft matrix
cultured epithelial autograft
cymba conchal cartilage g.
Cymetra tissue replacement
g.
Dardik Biograft vein g.
Diastat vascular access g.

graft (*continued*)
>   Distaflo bypass g.
>   DualMesh biomaterial
>   DuraGen g.
>   Durapatite g.
>   Edwards woven Teflon
>   aortic bifurcation g.
>   EpiFilm g.
>   Favaloro saphenous vein
>   bypass g.
>   Fluoropassiv thin-wall
>   carotid patch g.
>   Golaski g.
>   Grafton bone g.
>   Hapset hydroxyapatite bone
>   graft plaster
>   Healos bone g. substitute
>   material
>   Hedrocel bone substitute
>   material
>   Hemashield
>   HTO Wedge tissue allograft
>   H. Vantage g.
>   InterGard heparin vascular g.
>   InterPore g.
>   Ionescu-Shiley pericardial
>   xenograft
>   Kimura cartilage g.
>   MD-111 bone allograft
>   Meadox Microvel arterial g.
>   Microknit vascular g.
>   MycroMesh biomaterial
>   Paritene mesh
>   Perma-Flow coronary
>   bypass g.
>   PermaMesh
>   PermaSeal dialysis access g.
>   porcine xenograft
>   ProOsteon 500 bone
>   implant
>   Proplast g.
>   PTFE endovascular g.
>   Rapidgraft arterial vessel
>   substitute
>   Sauvage g.
>   Solvang g.
>   Sperma-Tex preshaped
>   mesh

graft (*continued*)
>   Surgipro prolene mesh
>   SurgiSis mesh
>   Thoralon biomaterial
>   TransCyte skin substitute
>   Trelex mesh
>   Unigraft bone graft material
>   Unilab Surgibone
>   Vascu-Guard bovine
>   pericardial surgical patch
>   Vascutek Gelseal vascular g.
>   Vectra vascular access
>   Venaflow vascular g.
>   Weaveknit vascular g.
>   Wesolowski vascular g.
>   XenoDerm g.
>   Zenith AAA endovascular g.
>   Zenotech g.

GraftAssist vein graft holder

Graftskin

Grams
>   G. nylon nonabsorbable
>   suture
>   G. polypropylene
>   nonabsorbable s.
>   G. silk nonabsorbable s.

grasper
>   Glassman g.

Gray bone drill

Greenwald
>   G. cutting loop
>   G. flexible endoscopic
>   electrodes

Grieshaber manipulator

Grosse and Kempf locking nail
>   system

Guardwire angioplasty system

Guglielmi Detachable Coil

guidewire (*spelled also* guide
>   wire)
>   ACS HI-Torque Balance
>   Middleweight g.

guidewire (*continued*)
  Athlete coronary g.
  Bard Commander PTCA g.
  Bentson g.
  Conceptus Robust g.
  Extra Sport coronary g.
  FasTrac g.
  FlexFinder g.
  floppy g.
  FloWire Doppler g.
  Geenan Endotorque g.
  HyTek g.
  Intercept-Vascular g.
  Lumina g.
  Lunderquist g.
  Magnum g.
  Microvasive Glidewire
  Mirage g.
  Mustang steerable g.
  Phantom cardiac g.
  QuickSilver hydrophilic-
    coated g.
  Prima laser g.
  Radiofocus Glidewire
  Silk g.

guidewire (*continued*)
  SilverSpeed hydrophilic g.
  Sniper Elite hydrophilic g.
  steerable guide wire system
  Storq g.
  Terumo g.
  TherOx infusion g.
  TomCat PTCA g.
  Ultra-Select g.
  VascuLink vascular access
    g.
  VertiGraft textured allograft
    bone g.
  WaveWire g.
  Whisper g.
  Zebra exchange g.

Gunther Tulip vena cava MRI
  filter

Gynex
  G. angle hook
  G. Emmett tenaculum
  G. endospeculum
  G. extended-reach needle
  G. iris hook

H

Haemonetics Cell Saver 5

Haid
  H. cervical plate
  H. Universal bone plate
    system

Hakim-Cordis pump

Hall
  H. air drill
  H. arthrotome
  H. bone bur
  H. dermatome
  H. mastoid bur
  H. Micro-Aire drill
  H. Neurairtome drill
  H. Orthairtome d.
  H. Osteon drill
  H. sacral anchor
  H. spinal screw
  H. Surgairtome d.
  H. valve
  H. valvulotome
  H. Versipower oscillating
    saw

Hammer mini-tubular external
  fixation system

Hancke/Vilmann biopsy handle
  instrument

HandPort hand-assist device

HandTact instrument set

Hansatome microkeratome

Harrington
  H. bladder retractor
  H. clamp forceps
  H. distraction
    instrumentation
  H. hook clamp
  H. pedicle hook
  H. spinal elevator
  H. spreader
  H. strut
  H. thoracic forceps
  H. vulsellum forceps

Harrison-Nicolle polypropylene
  pegs

Hartmann
  H. adenoidal curette
  H. alligator forceps
  H. clamp
  H. eustachian catheter
  H. hemostat
  H. knife
  H. nasal conchotome
  H. nasal-cutting forceps
  H. nasal speculum
  H. tonsillar dissector
  H. uterine biopsy
    forceps

Hasson
  H. blunt-end cannula
  H. graspers
  H. laparoscope
  H. needle-nose forceps
  H. open laparoscopy
    cannula
  H. retractor
  H. trocar
  H. uterine manipulator

Hastings frame

Haverhill dermal abrader

Heartflo automated anastomosis
  system

HeatProbe water
  irrigation/lavage system

Hecht fascia lata forceps

heliX knot pusher

Hemaflex PTCA sheath with
  obturator

Hemaquet PTCA sheath with
  obturator

Hemaseel
  H. APR fibrin sealant
  H. HMN

Hemobahn endovascular prosthesis

Hemoclip

hemostat
    Actifoam h.
    Allis h.
    Avitene Ultrafoam collagen h.
    Avtifoam active h.
    Blohmka tonsillar h.
    Boettcher h.
    Collastat OBP microfibrillar collagen h.
    Endo-Avitene microfibrillar collagen h.
    Gutglass h.
    Halsted mosquito h.
    Hartmann h.
    Hemaflex pure collagen h.
    hemostatic eraser
    Hemotene
    Nu-Knit absorbable h.

HepatAssist bioartificial liver

Herloon hernia balloon trocar

HerniaMesh
    H. surgical mesh
    H. surgical plug

Hersh
    H. LASIK retreatment forceps
    H. LASIK retreatment spatula

Hex-Fix fracture fixation system

Heyer-Schulte tissue expander

Hi-Torque
    H.-T. Flex-T guidewire
    H.-T. Floppy exchange guidfewire
    H.-T. Floppy with Pro/Pel
    H.-T. Standard guidewire

Hoek-Bowen cement removal system

Hoffmann
    H. external fixation device
    H. mini-lengthening fixation device

holder
    A-1-Askari needle h.
    Abbey needle h.
    Anis-Barraquer needle h.
    Arruga needle h.
    Azar needle h.
    Barraquer curved h.
    Baum-Metzenbaum sternal needle h.
    bladebreaker h.
    Bodkin thread h.
    Bozeman-Finochietto needle h.
    Bozeman-Wertheim needle h.
    Charnley trochanter h.
    Clerf needle h.
    Cottle needle h.
    DeBakey Vital needle h.
    Derlacki ossicle h.
    Endo-Assist disposable needle h.
    Giannini needle h.
    GraftAssist vein and graft h.
    House-Urban temporal bone h.
    Huang vein h.
    I-tech needle h.
    Jako laryngeal needle h.
    Jarcho tenaculum h.
    Jarit forceps h.
    Langenbeck needle h.
    Malis needle h.
    Millin boomerang needle h.
    Paparella monkey-head h.
    Rhoton bayonet needle h.
    Sinskey needle h.
    Stratte needle h.
    SurgiAssist surgical leg h.
    Tennant eye needle h.
    Tru-Cut biopsy needle h.
    Vital-Cooley French-eye needle h.

holder (*continued*)
  Vital-Neivert needle h.
  Watanabe pin h.
  Wehbe arm h.
  Yarsargil bayonet needle h.
  Zollinger leg h.
  Zweifel needle h.

hook
  Abramson h.
  boat h.
  Doyen rib h.
  Gillies h.
  Gynex angle h.
  Hirschman iris h.
  Isola spinal implant system h.
  Kelman manipulator h.
  Krayenbuehl nerve h.
  Mayo fibroid h.
  Miya h.
  Ochsner h.
  Pucci-Seed h.
  Rappazzo iris h.
  Rhoton nerve h.
  Russian four-pronged fixation h.
  Scoville curved nerve h.
  Sinskey iris h.
  Smithwick h.
  Storz iris h.
  Visitec double iris h.
  von Graefe muscle h.
  Zoellner h.

Hotsy Cautery

Howard corneal abrader

Howmedica
  H. Centrax head replacement
  H. cerclage
  H. Duracon implant
  H. Kinematic II knee prosthesis
  H. monotube
  H. Simplex P. cement
  H. Unitrax hip fracture system

Hulka
  H. clip
  H. tenaculum
  H. uterine cannula

HUMI uterine manipulator/catheter

Hummingbird wand

Hunter-Sessions balloon

hysteroscope
  ACMI Micro-H. h.
  AMSCO h.
  Baggish h.
  Baloser h.
  Elmed h.
  Fujinon flexible h.
  Galileo rigid h.
  Hamou h.
  Storz h.
  Valle h.

hydrokeratome

HydroThermAblator system

Hypergel

I-Flow nerve block infusion kit

Iglesias
- I. continuous-flow resectoscope
- I. dilator
- I. electrode
- I. evacuator
- I. fiberoptic resectoscope
- I. microlens resectoscope

Ilizarov
- I. circular external fixator
- I. distractor
- I. limb-lengthening system
- I. screw

Illi intracranial fixation device

Imagyn microlaparoscope

Immix bioabsorbable implant

Imount instruments

implant
- Acticon neosphincter i.
- Alpha 1 penile i.
- Arenberg-Denver inner-ear valve
- Baerveldt glaucoma i.
- Biocell RTV saline-filled breast i.
- Biocoral i.
- Biodel i.
- Bio-eye i.
- Biomatrix ocular i.
- Bionix SmartNail bioresorbable i.
- Branemark endosteal i.
- Clarion multi-strategy cochlear i.
- Codere orbital floor i.
- collagen meniscus i.
- Compliant pre-stress bone i.
- Contigen Bard cochlear i.
- Durapatite i.
- Heyer-Schulte i.
- IMEX scleral i.

implant (*continued*)
- Integral Omniloc i.
- Interpore i.
- Kerato-Gel i.
- Kinetik great toe i.
- McGhan facial i.
- Nexus i.
- NovaGold breast i.
- SoftForm facial i.
- Trilucent breast i.
- Unilab Surgibone i.
- Vitrasert intraocular i.

Incardia coronary artery bypass graft system

INCERT adhesion barrier

incision
- Bevan i.
- Bruser i.
- Cherney i.
- chevron i.
- gull-wing i.
- Kocher collar i.
- LaRoque herniorrhaphy i.
- Rethi i.
- Wilde i.
- Y i.
- Yorke-Mason i.

Indermil tissue adhesive

In-Fast bone screw system

InFix interbody fusion system

InjecTx cystoscope

InnovaTome microkeratome device

INRO surgical nail

Insall/Burstein II knee replacement system

InstaTrak endoscopic sinus surgery device

InStent
- I. balloon-expandable stent

InStent (*continued*)
    I. CarotidCoil stent

InSurg
    I. laparoscopic stone basket
    I. LapTie needle diver
       suturing device
    I. Pursuer CBD basket
    I. Segura CBD basket

In-Tac bone anchor

Integrity AFx pacemaker

Interax total knee system

Interceed adhesion barrier

Intercept vascular guidewire

Inter Fix spinal fusion cage

InterGard collagen graft

Inter-Op acetabular prosthesis

Intrafix tibial fastener

IntraStent biliary stent

introducer
    Allen spherical eye i.
    Angestat hemostasis i.
    Avanti i.
    Check-Flo i.
    Cook Peel-Away i.
    Desilets i.
    Encapsulon sheath i.
    Eschmann endotracheal
      tube i.
    Excalibur i.
    FasTrac i.
    Hedwig i.
    Hemaquet i.
    Intro Deuce double-lumen i.
    Nottingham i.
    Razi cannula i.
    Speck i.
    Tuohy-Borst side-arm i.
    Weaver trocar i.

introducer (*continued*)
    Wellwood-Ferguson i.

Ioban antimicrobial incise
   drape

Iodoflex absorptive dressing

iodoform gauze

iodophor Steri-drape

Iodosorb absorptive dressing

Ionescu-Shiley
    I.-S. artificial cardiac valve
    I.-S. pericardial valve
    I.-S. vascular graft

Iotec trocar

irrigator
    Baumrucker clamp i.
    Carabelli i.
    DeVilbiss eye i.
    Fisch bone drill i.
    Fluvog i.
    HydroSurg laparoscopic i.
    Irrijet i.
    Kelman i.
    LASIK flap i.
    Moncrieff anterior chamber
      i.
    Nezhat i.
    Ortholav pulsed i.
    Rollet anterior chamber i.
    Shambaugh i.
    Stopko i.
    Stryker suction i.
    Thornwald antral i.
    Vidaurri i.
    Younge i.
    Zerowet splash shield i.
    Zimmer suction i.

ISI laparoscopic instruments

Isola spinal instrumentation
   system

J

Jackson spinal surgery table

Jako
- J. knot pusher
- J. laryngeal suction tube
- J. laser retractor
- J. microlaryngeal grasping forceps
- J. suction tube

Jako-Kleinsasser
- J.-K. knife
- J.-K. microscissors

Jamshidi
- J. adult needle
- J. liver biopsy needle

Jamshidi-Kormed bone marrow biopsy needle

Jarcho
- J. self-retaining uterine cannula
- J. tenaculum forceps
- J. uterine tenaculum

Jelco
- J. intravenous catheter
- J. needle

Jelenko
- J. arch bars
- J. facial fracture appliance
- J. pliers
- J. splint

Jeter lag screw

Jocath Maestro coronary balloon catheter

Jography angiographic catheter

Joguide coronary guiding catheter

Jostent coronary stent graft

Judet
- J. dissector
- J. hip prosthesis
- J. impactor

J-Vac
- J. catheter
- J. closed wound drainage system
- J. drain

K

Kaltostat wound packing

KAM Super Sucker arthroscopic suction device

Kaneda anterior spine stabilizing device

Kantor-Berci video laryngoscope

Kappa pacemaker

Karickhoff laser lens

Kartush tympanic membrane patcher

Kasai peritoneal venous shunt

Katena cannula

K-Blade
    K. keratome
    K. super-sharp blade

keratome
    HydroBlade k.
    HydroBrush k.
    SatinSlit k.

Killian-Lynch laryngoscope

Killip wire

Kim-Ray Greenfield caval filter

Kitano knot

Kittner dissector

Kleinsasser anterior commissure larungoscope

knife
    Abraham tonsillar k.
    bladebraker k.

knife (*continued*)
    Cyberknife
    EdgeAhead phaco slit k.
    Foerster capsulotomy k.
    Freedom k.
    Harmonic scalpel
    Lebsche k.
    Neoflex bendable k.
    Parasmilllie k.
    Paufique k.
    ShortCut k.
    sickle k.
    Tiemann Meals tenolysis k.
    UltraCision ultrasonic k.
    Visitec circular k.
    Visitec crescent k.
    Visitec stiletto k.

Knifelight
    K. surgical knife
    K. surgical light

knot
    Aberdeen k.
    k. pusher
    k. tier

Koala vascular clamp

Koch phaco manipulator/ splitter

Kostuik internal spine fixation system

Kraff nucleus splitter

Kraff-Utrata tear capsulotomy forceps

Kugel hernia patch

L

Laborde
- L. dilator
- L. forceps

LactoSorb
- L. plating system
- L. resorbable craniomaxillofacial fixation
- L. resorbable fixation device

Ladd
- L. calipers
- L. elevator
- L. intracranial pressor sensor
- L. knife
- L. lid clamp

LaForce
- L. adenotome
- L. adenotome blade
- L. hemostatic tonsillectome

LaForce-Grieshaber adenotome

LaForce-Stevenson adenotome

LaForce-Storz adenotome

Lahey
- L. arterial forceps
- L. bronchial clamp
- L. drain
- L. gall duct forceps
- L. goiter retractor
- L. hemostat
- L. ligature passer
- L. needle
- L. operating scissors
- L. thyroid clamp
- L. thyroid scissors
- L. tenaculum forceps

lamp
- Alzheimer l.
- Birch-Hirschfeld l.
- Campbell slit l.

lamp (*continued*)
- Coherent LaserLink slit l.
- Duke-Elder l.
- Faro coolbeam l.
- Grafco perineal l.
- Ishihara IV slit l.
- Marco slit l.
- Posner slit l.
- Rodenstock slit l.
- Thorpe slit l.
- Wood l.
- Zeiss carbon arc slit l.

Lane
- L. bone-holding clamp
- L. bone screw
- L. cleft palate needle
- L. fasciatome
- L. gastrointestinal forceps
- L. mouth gag
- L. screwdriver
- L. tissue forceps

LaparoLift system

LaparoSAC
- L. single-use cannula
- L. single-use obturator

laparoscope
- ACMI Transvaginal Hydro l.
- Circon ACMI diagnostic l.
- Dyonics rod lens l.
- Elmed diagnostic l.
- Frangenheim l.
- Fujinon diagnostic l.
- Hasson l.
- Kuda l.
- MiniSite l.
- Polaris l.
- Ruddock l.
- Sharplav l.
- Stoltz l.
- Storz diagnostic l.
- Storz operating l.
- Surgiview multi-use disposable l.

laparoscope (*continued*)
    Wolf insufflation l.
    Ziskie operating l.

Laparosonic coagulating shears

Lap-Band adjustable gastric
    banding system

Lapides
    L. catheter
    L. holder
    L. needle

Lapro-Clip

LapTie endoscopic knot-tying
    instrument

Lap Vacu-Irrigator

Lapwall laparotomy sponge

laryngoscope
    Bullard intubating l.
    Chevalaier Jackson l.
    Clerf l.
    Dedo-Jako l.
    Dedo laser l.
    Flexiblade l.
    Holinger l.
    Hollister l.
    Jackson l.
    Jako l.
    Killian-Lynch suspension l.
    Kleinsasser operating l.
    Lewy anterior commissure l.
    Lewy suspension l.
    Lindholm operating l.
    Machida fiberoptic l.
    Magill l.
    NLite l.
    Ossloff-Karlan-Dedo l.
    Ossloff-Karlan-Jako l.
    Ossloff-Karlan laser l.
    Rusch l.
    Storz-Hopkins l.
    Storz-Riecker l.
    Tucker anterior
        commissure l.
    Weerda distending
        operating l.

laryngoscope (*continued*)
    Welch Allyn l.
    Yankauer l.

laser
    AccuLase excimer l.
    AcuBlade robotic l.
    alexandrite l.
    Arago argon l.
    ArF excimer l.
    argon/krypton l.
    Athos l.
    ArthroProbe l.
    Aurora diode l.
    Aurora HL l.
    Candela 405-mm pulsed
        dye l.
    CHRYS CO2 l.
    Cilco argon l.
    ClearView CO2 l.
    CO2 Heart Laser 2 l.
    Coherent CO2 surgical l.
    Coherent Selectra 7000 l.
    Coherent UltraPulse 5000C
        l.
    Coherent Versapulse
    CoolGlide l.
    Cooper LaserSonics l.
    CooperVision argon l.
    copper-vapor pulsed l.
    Crystalase erbium l.
    Derma K l.
    DermaLase l.
    DioLite l.
    Diomed surgical diode l.
    Dodick l. Photolysis system
    Eclipse TMR l.
    EpiLaser
    EpiStar diode l.
    EpiTouch
    FCP2 l.
    FeatherTouch CO_2 l.
    Fiberlase l.
    Flashlamp-pulsed Nd:YAG l.
    Flexlase 600 l.
    GentleLASE Plus l.
    GyneLase diode l.
    Heart Laser

laser (*continued*)
Hoskins nylon suture laser l.
Hyperion LTK l.
Kaplan PenduLaser surgical l.
Kirsch l.
Kremer excimer l.
krypton (red) l.
LADARVision excimer l.
Lambda Plus dye l.
LaserHarmonic l.
Laser Lancet l.
LaserSonics l.
Nidek EC-5000 excimer l.
NovaLine Litho-S DUV excimer l.
NovaPulse CO_2 l.
Novulase 660 l.
PhotoGenica V-Star l.
Q-LAS 10 YAG l.
Opmilas CO_2 l.
Pegasus Nd:YAG surgical l.
Prostalase l.
PulseMaster l.
Q-switched ruby l.
ScleroLaser
ScleroPlus
SilkLaser l.
Smoothbeam l.
Surgilase Nd:YAG l.
SurgiLight OptiVision YAG l.
Topaz CO_2 l.
TruPulse CO_2 l.
UltraFine erbium l.
UltraPulse CO_2 l.
Urolase fiber l.
VersaLight l.
VersaPulse holmium l.
Visulas Hd:YAG l.
VISX excimer l.
VISX Star S2 excimer l.
Waterlase Millennium l.
XTRAC l. system
Zeiss Visulas 690 l.
Zyoptix l.

Lasermedic Microlight 830

LaserPen

LaserSonics
L. EndoBlade
L. Nd:YAG LaserBlade scalpel
L. SurgiBlade

Lawrence
L. Add-A-Cath
L. deep forceps
L. hemostatic forceps

lead
Accufix pacemaker l.
Aescula
AngeFlex l.
Attain steroid-eluting l.
Biotronik l.
CapSure cardiac pacing l.

LeBag ileocolic urinary reservoir

LeFort
L. dilator
L. filiform
L. filiform bougie
L. speculum
L. suture
L. urethral sound
L. uterine sound

Leibinger
L. Micro Dynamic Mesh
L. miniplate system
L. Profyle system
L. Würzburg plate

lens
Abraham contact l.
Abraham iridectomy laser l.
Abraham peripheral button iridotomy l.
Abraham YAG laser l.
AcrySof foldable intraocular l.
Adaptar contact l.
AMO Array foldable intraocular l.
AMO Sensar posterior chamber intraocular l.
Array multifocal intraocular l.

lens (*continued*)
Artisan phakic intraocular l.
Bagolini l.
Baikoff l.
Baron l.
CeeOn heparinized
intraocular l.
Cilco Slant l.
Coburn equiconvex l.
Collamer one-piece l.
Dulaney intraocular implant
l.
etafilcon A. l.
Focus Night & Day contact l.
Foroblique l.
Galand disc l.
Goldmann l.
Hoskins nylon suture laser l.
Hruby l.
Hydroview intraocular l.
IOLAB Slimfit l.
Karickhoff laser l.
Kelman intraocular l.
Leiske l.
Leib-Guerry cataract
implant l.
Mainster retina laser l.
MemoryLens
Monoflex l.
Morgan l.
PhacoFlex l.
PMMA contact l.
Prokop intraocular l.
SeeQuence disposable l.
Silsoft extended wear
contact l.
SingleStitch PhacoFlex l.
Slant l.
Staar foldable
intraocular l.
Volk pan retinal l.
Worst gonioprism
contact l.

LeVeen peritoneal shunt

Lexer
L. chisel
L. dissecting scissors

Lexer (*continued*)
L. gouge
L. osteotome
L. tissue forceps

LifeSite hemodialysis access
system

Ligaclip

ligature
l. cannula
Desault l.
Potts l.
Surgiwip suture l.
l. tie wire

Lindstrom arcuate incision
marker

Link
L. cementless hip
prosthesis
L. Endo-Model rotational
knee prosthesis
L. Lubinus SP II hip
prosthesis
L. Stack Split splint

Linvatec
L. absorbable screw
L. Advantage shaver
L. cannula
L. driver
L. Lightning blade resector
L. meniscal BioStinger
anchor suture

lithotripter
Breakstone l.
Calcutript l.
Dormia gallstone l.
Dornier waterbath l.
Genestone 190 l.
Lithoclast l.
Lithostar l.
Medstone STS l.
Modulith SL 20 l.
Piezolith-EPL l.
Pulsolith l.
Sonolith Praktis l.
Storz Monolith l.

Livernois lens-holding forceps

Livernois-McDonald forceps

LoPro right angle ArthroWand

Lord total hip prosthesis

Luhr
- L. fixation plate
- L. microbone plate
- L. minifixation bone plate
- L. Vitallium micromesh plate
- L. Vitallium screw

Luminexx biliary stent

Luque
- L. cerclage wire
- L. L-rod
- L. rod
- L. semirigid segmental spinal instrumentation
- L. sublaminar wire

Lusk instrument

Luxtec
- L. fiberoptic system
- L. Surgical telescope

lyodura loop

M

McCutchen
   M. press-fit titanium
     femoral implant
   M. SLT hip prosthesis

McDonald
   M. bone plate
   M. cerclage
   M. dissector
   M. gastric clamp
   M. lens-folding forceps

McDougal prostatectomy clamp

McGhan
   M. breast implant
   M. eye implant
   M. facial implant
   M. lens
   M. plastic surgical needle
   M. tissue expander

McGlamry elevator

Machida
   M. fiberoptic laryngoscope
   M. light source connector

Maciol laparoscopic suture
  needle set

McPherson
   M. angled forceps
   M. bent forceps
   M. eye speculum
   M. Irrigating forceps
   M. straight bipolar forceps
   M. trabeculotome
   M. tying iris forceps

Macroplastique bulking agent

MacroPore OS spinal system

Madayag biopsy needle

Maestro bipolar dual-chamber
  pacemaker

Magic
   M. microcatheter
   M. Torque guidewire

Malecot
   M. four-wing catheter
   M. nephrostomy catheter
   M. reentry catheter
   M. Silastic catheter
   M. suprapubic cystostomy
     catheter

Malis
   M. angled bayonet forceps
   M. bipolar coagulation
     forceps
   M. cerebellar retractor
   M. clip applier
   M. CMC-II bipolar
     coagulator
   M. dissector
   M. hinge clamp
   M. irrigation forceps
   M. ligature passer
   M. nerve hook
   M. neurosurgical scissors

Mallinckrodt
   M. angiographic catheter
   M. endotracheal tube
   M. Laser-Flex tube
   M. vertebral catheter

Malmstrom cup

manipulator
   Barrett flange lens m.
   ClearView uterine m.
   Drysdale nucleus m.
   Feaster lens m.
   Grieshaber three-function m.
   Guimaraes implantable
     contact lens m.
   Hasson uterine m.
   Hirschman lens m.
   Hulka uterine m.
   Koch phaco .
   Kuglen angled lens m.
   Pelosi uterine m.
   Rappazzo intraocular m.
   RUMI uterine m.
   ZUMI uterine m.

MAPcath stylet

MAPwire J-tip guidewire

Mark
M. II Chandler retractor
M. II Kodros radiolucent
awl

marker
Amsler scleral m.
Arrowsmith corneal m.
Castroviejo scleral m.
Dulaney LASIK m.
Feldman radial
keratotomu m.
Freeman cookie cutter
areola m.
Gonin-Amsler scleral m.
Hoopes corneal m.
Lundstrom arcuate
incision m.
Machat superior flap
LASIK m.
Nordan-Ruiz trapezoidal m.
Price radial m.
Saunders-Paparella m.
Simcoe corneal m.
Skin Skribe m.
Storz radial incision m.
TLS surgical m.
Vismark surgical skin m.

Marlex
M. band
M. mesh
M. mesh graft
M. methyl methacrylate
prosthesis
M. methyl methacrylate
sandwich
M. Perfix plug
M. suture

Maryland dissector

material
Apligraf skin graft m.
Biobrane/HF graft m.
Bioglass bone
substitute m.

material (*continued*)
Biograft bovine heterograft
m.
Bioplastique augmentation,
m.
Biovert implant m.
Carbo-Seal graft m.
Carbo-Zinc skin barrier m.
Celestin graft m.
Codman cranioplastic m.
Collagraft bone graft matrix
m.
DermAssist wound filling m.
Dextran-70 barrier m.
Durapatite bone
replacement m.
Epicel skin graft m.
FlowGel barrier m.
Gore-Tex alloplastic m.
Grafton bone grafting m.
Healos synthetic bone
grafting m.
Interceed barrier m.
Interpore bone
replacement m.
MycroMesh graft m.
OsteoGraf bone grafting m.
PolyWic wound filling m.
ProOsteon implant graft m.
SeamGuard staple line m.
Surgical Nu-Knit absorbable
hemostatic m.
Zenotech graft m.

May
M. bone plate
M. kidney clamp

Mayfield
M. aneurysm clamp
M. bayonet osteotome
M. CIS-RE aneurysm clamp
M. clip applicator
M. fixation frame
M. head clamp
M. malleable brain spatula
M. pediatric horseshoe
headrest
M. retractor

Mayfield (*continued*)
M. skull clamp pin
M. spinal curette
M. tic headholder
M.-Kees clip
M.-Kees headholder
M.-Kees skull fixation
apparatus
M.-Kees table attachment

Mayo
M. abdominal retractor
M. common duct probe
M. cystic duct scoop
M. Fibroid hook
M. gallstone scoop
M. kidney clamp
M. linen suture
M. operating scissors
M. round blade scissors
M. tissue forceps
M. trocar needle
M. uterine probe
M. uterine scissors
M. vessel clamp

Medicon
M. instruments
M. rib retractor
M. ultrasonic liposuction
device
M. wire-twister forceps

Medi-Tech
M. arterial dilatation
catheter
M. guidewire
M. IVC filter
M. multipurpose basket
M. occlusion balloon
catheter
M. steerable catheter
M. stone basket
M. wire

MedJet microkeratome

Mednext bone dissecting
system

Medoff sliding fracture plate

Medtronic
M. AneuRx stent graft
M. AVE S660 coronary stent
M. BeStent stent
M. bipolar pacemaker
M. cardiac cooling jacket
M. Cardiorhythm Atakr
generator
M. Chardack pacemaker
M. ClearCut 2
electrosurgical handpiece
M. Elite II pacemaker
M Gem automatic
implantable defibrillator
M. Hemopump
M. Inspire system
M. Micro Jewel defibrillator
M. Minix pacemaker
M. Octopus
M. Pacette pacemaker
M. Spirit lead
M. SPO pacemaker
M. Symbios pacemaker
M. SynchroMed implantable
pump
M. Thera i-series cardiac
pacemaker
M. Transvene endocardial
lead
M. Zuma guiding catheter
M.-Alcatel pacemaker
M.-Byrel-SX pacemaker

Mefilm dressing

MegaLink biliary stent

Melgisorb calcium alginate
dressing

membrane
barrier m.
biobarrier m.
BioGen nonporous barrier
m.
Bio-Gide resorbable barrier
m.
BioMend collagen m.
Biopore m.
Hemophan m.

Onlay patch

membrane (*continued*)
    Imtec BioBarrier m.
    m. peeler
    Preclude pericardial m.
    Preclude peritoneal m.
    Preclude spinal m.
    Seprafilm
      bioresorbable m.

Memotherm
    M. colorectal stent
    M. endoscopic biliary stent
    M. Flexx biliary stent
    M. nitinol stent

meniscotome
    Drompp m.
    Dyonics m.
    Grover m.
    Ruuska m.
    Smillie m.

Mentor
    M. absorbent pouch
    M. biliary stent
    M. breast prosthesis
    M. coude catheter
    M. Foley catheter
    M. IPP penile prosthesis
    M. prostate biopsy needle
    M. straight catheter
    M. tissue expander
    M. Wet-Field cautery

Mepiform dressing

Mepilex foam dessing

Mepitel dressing

Mepore absorptive dressing

Merocel
    M. epistaxis packing
    M. sponge
    M. surgical spear
    M. tampon

Merogel
    M. dressing
    M. nasal packing
    M. stent

mesh
    Auto Suture surgical m.
    Bard-Marlex m.
    Bard Sperma-Tex
      preshaped m.
    Brennen biosynthetic
      surgical m.
    Composix m.
    craniomaxillofacial m.
    Dacron m.
    Dexon m.
    DualMesh m.
    Dumbach titanium m.
    FortaGen m.
    Herniamesh surgical m.
    Kugel m.
    Medox Dacron m.
    MycroMesh biomaterial
    Parietex composite m.
    PerFix Marlex m. plug
    Permacol m.
    Prolene m.
    Sepramesh biosurgical
      composite
    Surgipro hernia m.
    SynMesh m.
    Teflon m.
    ThermoFX m.
    TiMesh cranial m.
    TiMesh orbital m.
    TiMesh titanium m.
    Trelex natural m.
    Visilex polypropylene m.

Messerklinger sinus endoscopy
    set

MetraGrasp ligament
    grasper

MetraPass suture passer

MetraTie knot pusher

Metzenbaum
    M. chisel
    M. dissecting scissors
    M. gouge
    M. needle holder
    M. tonsillar forceps

MIC
  MIC gastroenteric tube
  MIC jejunal tube
  MIC jejunostomy tube

MIC-KEY gastrostomy tube

MicroBite forceps

Microblator small joint
  ArthroWand

MicroCAP ArthroWand

Micro Diamond-Point
  microsurgery instruments

MicroFrance
  M. minimally invasive
    surgical instruments
  M. pediatric backbiter

MicroGlide reciprocating
  osteotome

Microknit vascular graft
  prosthesis

MicroLap Gold
  microlaparoscope

Micron bobbin ventilation
  tube

Micropuncture peel-away
  introducer

MicroSmooth probe

Microvasive
  M. biliary stent
  M. Geenen Endotorque
    guide wire
  M. Glidewire
  M. One Step Button
    gastrostomy
  M. papillotome
  M. Rigiflex TTS balloon
  M. sclerotherapy needle
  M. Speedband Superview
    ligator
  M. stiff piano wire guide
    wire
  M. ultratome

Microvit
  M. cutter
  M. probe
  M. scissors
  M. vitrector

Miltex surgical instruments

Mitek
  M. anchor
  M. Fastin threaded anchor
  M. Knotless anchor suture
  M. Ligament anchor
  M. Micro QuickAnchor
  M. Panalot anchor
  M. suture
  M. Tacit threaded anchor
  M. Vapr tissue removal
    system

Mitraflex wound dressing

Mixter
  M. arterial forceps
  M. common duct probe
  M. gallbladder forceps
  M. mosquito forceps
  M. thoracic clamp
  M. ventricular needle

Miya hook ligament carrier

Mobin-Uddin umbrella filter

Modulap cutting and
  coagulating probe

Molnar disk

Monoscopy locking trocar

Monticelli-Spinelli system

Moolgaoker forceps

Moretz Tab ventilation tube

Morscher titanium cervical plate

Morse
  M. blade
  M. sternal retractor
  M. suction tube
  M. taper stem
  M. towel clip
  M. valve retractor

Moss
- M. balloon triple-lumen gastrostomy tube
- M. cage
- M. G-tube PEG kit
- M. hook
- M. Mark IV tube
- M. Miami load-sharing spinal implant system
- M. nasal tube
- M. rod
- M. Suction Buster tube
- M. T-anchor needle introducer gun

MPC scissors

MPort foldable lens placement system

Mueller
- M. aortic clamp
- M. bur
- M. catheter
- M. curette
- M. electric corneal trephine
- M. eye speculum

Mueller (*continued*)
- M. forceps
- M. lacrimal sac retractor
- M. needle
- M. pediatric clamp
- M. saw
- M. total hip prosthesis
- M. vena cava clamp

Multibite biopsy forceps

Multiclip

Multi-Link
- M. coronary stent system
- M. Penta stent
- M. Pixel stent
- M. Tetra coronary stent

Multispatula cervical sampling device

Multitak suture system

MultiVac
- M. TriStar ArthroWand
- M. XL ArthroWand

N

nail
Albizzia n.
Bickel intramedullary n.
Biomet ankle arthrodesis n.
Brooker-Wills n.
Dooley n.
Gamma trochanteric
locking n.
Grosse-Kempf femoral n.
Hagie pin n.
Hahn bone n.
Harris hip n.
IMSC five-hole n.
Inro surgical n.
intramedullary skeletal
kinetic distractor n. (ISKD)
Jewett hip n.
Koslowski hip n.
Massie sliding n.
Moore adjustable n.
Nylok self-locking n.
Orthofix intramedullary n.
Palmer bone n.
Recon n.
Sampson fluted n.
Seidel humeral locking n.
Smillie n.
Staples osteotomy n.
Steinmann extension n.
Synthes titanium elastic n.
Uniflex intramedullary n.
Vitallium n.
Z-fixation n.
Zickel n.
Zimmer telescoping n.

Nakao
N. Ejector biopsy forceps
N. snare

Navigator flexible endoscope

Naviport deflectable tip guiding
catheter

needle
Abrahms biopsy n.
Abscession n.

needle (*continued*)
Accucore II biopsy n.
Ailee n.
arachnophlebectomy n.
Atraloc surgical n.
BD SafetyGlide n.
Bierman n.
Biopty cut n.
BRK transseptal n.
Brockenbrough n.
Cardiopoint n.
Charles flute n.
Chiba n.
Cibis ski n.
CIF-4 n.
coaxial sheath cut-biopsy n.
Cobb-Ragde n.
Colapinto n.
Concept suturing n.
Control-Release pop-off n.
Cook endoscopic curved n.
driver
Core aspiration/injection n.
Core CO_2 insufflation n.
DeBakey n.
Dieckmann intraosseous n.
D-Tach removable n.
Dos Santos n.
Echo-Coat ultrasound
biopsy n.
Endopath Ultra Veress n.
Ethalloy TruTaper n.
Franseen n.
French-eye n.
Goldenberg Snarecoil bone
marrow biopsy n.
GraNee n.
Hawkeye suture n.
Hawkins breast localization
n.
Howell biopsy aspiration n.
Huber n.
Impex aspiration and
injection n.
Injex disposable n.
IOLAB taper-cut n.

needle (*continued*)
    J n.
    Jamshidi-Kormed bone
        marrow biopsy n.
    Jamshidi liver biopsy n.
    Keith n.
    Klatskin liver biopsy n.
    Lewis Pair-Pak n.
    Madayag biopsy n.
    Mayo catgut n.
    Menghini liver biopsy n.
    MicroFlow
        phacoemulsification n.
    milliner's n.
    Nottingham
        colposuspension n.
    Osgood n.
    Ostycut bone biopsy n.
    ParaPRO paracentesis n.
    Pencan spinal n.
    PercuCut cut-biopsy n.
    Pereyra n.
    Plum-Blossom n.
    Protect Point n.
    Punctur-Guard n.
    Quantico n.
    Quincke spinal n.
    Riza-Ribe grasping n.
    Rosen n.
    Rosenthal n.
    Rycroft n.
    Saberloc spatula n.
    SafeTap tapered spinal n.
    Safety AV fistula n.
    Sahli n.
    SampleMaster biopsy n.
    Seldinger gastrostomy n.
    self-aspirating cut-biopsy n.
    Skinny n.
    SmallPort n.
    SmartNeedle
    Solitaire n.
    spatulated half-circle n.
    Stamey n.
    Steis n.
    Stifcore aspiration n.
    SuperGlide n.
    Terry-Mayo n.

THI n.
    Thomas n.
    Tru-Cut n.
    Tuohy n.
    Unimar J n.
    Visi-Black surgical n.
    Voorhees n.
    Waterfield n.
    Westerman-Jensen n.
    Whitacre spinal n.
    Wright n.

needle holder
    Dubecq-Princeteau
        angulating n. h.
    Nolan n. h.

Nélaton rubber tube drain

NeoKnife electrosurgical
    instrument

Neo-Sert umbilical vessel
    catheter

Neufeld
    N. device
    N. femoral nail plate
    N. nail
    N. pin
    N. screw
    N. traction

NeuroCol neurosurgical sponge

Neuroguide
    N. optical handpiece
    N. peel-away catheter
        introducer
    N. suction-irrigation adapter
    N. Visicath viewing catheter

NeuroMate sterotactic robot

Neuromeet
    N. nerve approximator
    N. universal soft tissue
        approximator

Neuro-Trace instrument

Neville-Barnes forceps

Nevyas drape retractor

Newvicon vacuum chamber pickup tube

NexGen complete knee replacement components

Nezhat-Dorsey Trumpet Valve hydrodissector

Nibbler device

Nibblit laparoscopic device

Nicola
    N. forceps
    N. gouge
    N. rasp
    N. tendon clamp

Niehaber prosthesis

NIR
    N. ON Ranger balloon expandable stent
    N. Primo Monorail stent system
    N. with SOX over-the-wire coronary stent system

Niroyal Elite Monorail coronary stent system

nitanol
    n. guidewire
    n. mesh-covered frame
    n. mesh stent
    n. self-expanding coil stent
    n. subglottic stenosis stent
    n. thermal memory stent

Noiles
    N. posterior stabilized knee prosthesis
    N. rotating hinge total knee prosthesis

NoProfile balloon catheter

Normigel hydrogel dressing

Normlgel protective wound dressing

No Sting barrier film

Novacor left ventricular assist system

NovaGold breast implant

NovaPulse CO_2 laser

NovaSaline inflatable breast implant

NovaSure endometrial ablation system

Novoste Beta-Cath system

Novus LC threaded interbody fusion cage

Nucleotome
    N. Endoflex instrument
    N Flex II cutting probe

Nuport PEG tube

Nu-Tip disposable scissor tip

NUVO barrier film

Nyhus/Nelson tube

Nylok self-locking nail

Oasis
  O. collagen plug
  O. feather microscalpel
  O. sheet introducer system
  O. thrombectomy system
  O. wound dressing

obturator
  Alcock o.
  blunt o.
  Cripps o.
  Ellik-Shaw o.
  Endotrac o.
  Fitch o.
  LaparoSAC o.
  Optiview optical surgical o.
  Thermafil Plus o.
  Timberlake o.
  ureteral catheter o.

Obwegeser
  O. awl
  O. channel retractor
  O. periosteal retractor
  O. splitting chisel
  O.-Dalpont internal screw
    fixation

Ochsner
  O. aortic clamp
  O. arterial forceps
  O. cartilage forceps
  O. Flexible spiral gallstone
    probe
  O. gallbladder tube
  O. hook
  O. needle
  O. ribbon retractor
  O. scissors
  O. thoracic clamp
  O. tissue/cartilage forceps
  O. vascular retractor
  O. wire twister

O'Connor
  O. biopsy forceps
  O. eye forceps
  O. grasping forceps

O'Connor (*continued*)
  O. iris forceps
  O. lid forceps
  O. marker
  O. muscle hook
  O. scleral depressor
  O. sheath
  O. sponge forceps
  O. vaginal retractor

Odyssey phacoemulsification
  system

Ogura
  O. cartilage forceps
  O. nasal saw
  O. tissue and cartilage
    forceps

Olatunbosun cerclage

Olympus
  O. CF-1T100L colonoscope
  O. CF-200Z colonoscope
  O. CYF-3OES
    cystofiberscope
  O. ENF-P2 flexible
    laryngoscope
  O. EVIS 140 endoscope
  O. EVIS Q-200V video
    endoscope
  O. FBK 13 endoscopic
    biopsy forceps
  O. GF-UM3 ultrasonic
    endoscope
  O. CF-UM20 ultrasonic
    endoscope
  O. GIF-EUM2
    echoendoscope
  O. GIF-1T10
    echoendoscope
  O. GIF-20 echoendoscope
  O. JF1T10 fiberoptic
    duodenoscope
  O. JF-UM20 echoendoscope
  O. One-Step button
  O. OSF flexible
    sigmoidoscope

Olympus (*continued*)
  O. SIF10 enteroscope
  O. TJF-100 endoscope
  O. UM-1W endoscopic
    probe
  O. URF-P2
    translaparoscopic
    choledochofiberscope
  O. VU-Ms echoendoscope
  O. XIF-UM3 echoendoscope
  O. XQ230 gastroscope

Omed bulldog vascular clamp

Ommaya
  O. intraventricular reservoir
    system
  O. retromastoid reservoir
  O. shunt
  O. spinal fluid reservoir
  O. ventricular tube

OmniCath atherectomy catheter

Omnifit
  O. acetabular cup
  O. HA femoral component
  O. HA hip stem
  O. intraocular lens
  O. knee prosthesis
  O. Plus offset cemented hip
    system

Omniflex
  O. balloon
  O. balloon catheter

OmniLink biliary stent

OmniStent stent

On-Command catheter

One-Shot anastomotic
  instrument

Opal tissue ablation device

Opera Star SL hysteroscope

Opmilas
  O. CO_2 multipurpose
    laser
  O. 144 Plus laser system

OpSite
  O. drape
  O. dressing
  O. Flexifix transparent film
    dressing
  O. Flexigrid adhesive film d.
  O. occlusive dressing
  O. PLUS dressing
  O. wound dressing

Optipore wound-cleaning
  sponge

Oracle
  O. Focus PTCA catheter
  O. Megasonics catheter
  O. Micro catheter
  O. Micro Plus PTCA
    catheter

Orbis-Sigma cerebrospinal fluid
  shunt valve

Oreopoulos-Zellerman catheter

Origin
  O. balloon
  O. tacker
  O. trocar

Orion
  O. anterior cervical plate
  O. balloon
  O. pacemaker
  O. plate and screw

Orthofix
  O. Cervical-Stim cervical
    bone growth stimulator
  O. external fixator
  O. intramedullary nail
  O. lengthening device
  O. pin
  O. screw

Ortho-Gen bone growth
  stimulator

Ortho-Glass cast material

Ortholoc
  O. Advantim knee revision
    system

Ortholoc (*continued*)
O. Advantim total knee system
O. prosthesis

OrthoNail intramedullary fixation device

OrthoPak II bone growth stimulator

Orthoplast
O. dressing
O. fracture brace
O. isoprene splint

Orthosorb absorbable pin

Osher
O. bipolar coaptation forceps
O. conjunctival forceps
O. corneal scissors
O. globe rotator
O. haptic forceps
O. iris retractor
O. lens-vacuuming cannula
O. malleable microspatula
O. needle holder
O. nucleus lens manipulator
O. nucleus stab expressor
O. superior rectus forceps

OssaTron orthotripsy

Ossoff-Karlan
O.-K. laser forceps
O.-K. laser laryngoscope
O.-K. laser suction tube
O.-K. microlaryngeal laser probe

Ossoff-Karlen laryngoscope

Osteo-Clage cerclage cable system

OsteoGen
O. bone graft
O. implantable stimulator

Osteogenics BoneSource synthetic bone replacement material

Osteomatrix bone filler

Osteon
O. bur
O. drill

Osteonics
O. acetabular dome hole plug
O.-HA coated implant
O. jig
O. Omnifit-HA hip stem
O. reamer
O. Scorpio insert
O. spinal system

Osteoset bone graft substitute

osteotome
Albee o.
Army o.
Barsky nasal o.
bayonet o.
Bowen o.
Box o
Carroll-Legg o.
Chermel o.
Cinelli o.
Cloward spinal fusion o.
Cobb o.
Codman o.
Cottle crossbar chisel o.
Dautery o.
Dingman o.
Epstein o.
Fomon o.
Furnas bayonet o.
Hlbbs o.
Hohmann o.
Hoke o.
Howorth o.
Jarit hand surgery o.
Kazanjian action-type o.
Lahey Clinic thin o.
Legg o.
Lexer o.
Manchester nasal o.

osteotome (*continued*)
  Mayfield bayonet o.
  Meyerding o.
  Micro-Aire o.
  Moberg o.
  Moe o.
  Neivert o.
  Padgett o.
  Parkes-Quisling o.
  Rhoton o.
  Rish o.
  Ristow o.
  Rubin nasofrontal o.
  Silver o.
  Stille o.
  Swanson o.
  Tardy o.
  Tessier o.
  Ward nasal o

O'Sullivan
  O.-O'Connor self-retaining
    abdominal retractor

O'Sullivan (*continued*)
  O.-O'Connor vaginal
    retractor
  O.-O'Connor vaginal
    speculum

Oto-Wick
  Pope O.

Overholt
  O. clip-applying forceps
  O. dissecting forceps
  O. periosteal elevator
  O. rib needle
  O. rib spreader

Oxiplex adhesive barrier

Oxiport blade

Oxycel
  O. dressing
  O. gauze

pacemaker
   AA1 single-chamber p.
   Accufix p
   Acculith p.
   Activitrax p.
   activity-guided p.
   activity-sensing p.
   Actros p.
   AddVent atrial-ventricular p.
   Affinity p.
   Atricor Cordis p.
   Autima II dual chamber p.
   Biotronic demand p.
   Chardack Medtronic p.
   Command PS p.
   Cordis Atricor p.
   Cordis Chronocor IV p.
   Cordis Ectocor P.
   Cordis Gemini cardiac p.
   Cordis Sequicor cardiac p.
   Cosmos II p.
   Dash p.
   Diamond II DDR p.
   Elite dual chamber rate-
      responsive p.
   Enterra p.
   Entity p.
   Ergos O_2 p.
   Fast-Pass lead p.
   Galaxy p.
   Genisis dual-chamber p.
   Guidant p.
   Intermedics Quantum
      unipolar p.
   Integrity AFx p.
   Jade II SSI p.
   Kairos p.
   Kappa p.
   Medtronic temporary p.
   Micro Minix p.
   Momentum p.
   Pacesetter Affinity p.
   Pacesetter Regency SC+ p.
   Pacesetter Synchrony p.
   Quantum p.
   Philos DR p.

pacemaker (*continued*)
   Relay cardiac p.
   Ruby II DDD p.
   SAVVI synchronous p.
   Topaz II SSIR p.
   Trilogy DC+ p.
   Trilogy SR+ p.
   Triumph VR p.
   Unity-C p.
   Ventak p.
   Vitatron Diamond II p.

Pacesetter
   P. AddVent 2060 LR p.
   P. Affinity pacemaker
   P. APS pacemaker
      programmer
   P. knee brace
   P. Regency SC+
      pacemaker
   P. Synchrony pacemaker
   P. Tendril DX steroid-eluting
      active-fixation pacing lead
   P. Trilogy DR+ pulse
      generator

Palmaz
   P. arterial stent
   P. balloon-expandable stent
   P. Corinthian transhepatic
      biliary stent
   P. vascular stent
   P.-Schatz balloon-
      expandable stent
   P.-Schatz biliary stent
   P.-Schatz Crown balloon-
      expandable stent
   P.-Schatz Mini Crown stent

Palmer
   P. biopsy forceps
   P. bone nail
   P. cruciate ligament guide
   P. cutting forceps
   P. grasping forceps
   P. lens
   P. ovarian biopsy forceps

Palmer (*continued*)
   P. uterine dilator

Panalok
   P. absorbable soft tissue
     anchor
   P. RC absorbable soft tissue
     anchor
   P. QuickAnchor Plus suture
     anchor

panendoscope
   cap-fitted p.
   flexible forward-
     viewing p.
   Foroblique p.
   LoPresti p.
   McCarthy p.
   Stern-McCarthy p.
   Storz p.
   Wolf rigid p.

Panje
   P. tube
   P. voice button

PanoGauze
   P. dressing
   P. hydrogel-impregnated
     gauze

PanoView
   P. arthroscopic system
   P. Optics lens
   P. rod-lens ureteroscope

Paparella
   P. angled-ring curette
   P. canal knife
   P. catheter
   P. duckbill elevator
   P. footplate pick
   P. mastoid curette
   P. myringotomy tube
   P. probe
   P. self-retaining retractor
   P. sickle knife
   P. stapes curette
   P. straight needle
   P. type II ventilation tuber
   P. wire-cutting scissors

papillotome
   Accuratome precurved p.
   Apollo 3 triple-lumen p.
   Bard Companion p.
   Bilisystem wire-guided p.
   Cremer-Ideda p.
   Erlangen p.
   Howell rotatable BII p.
   Microvasive p.
   needle-knife p.
   Piggyback needle-knife p.
   precut p.
   ProForma double-lumen p.
   shark fin p.
   Swenson p.
   Wilson-Cook p.
   Wiltek p.
   Zimmon p.

Parachute Corkscrew suture
   anchor

Paragon
   P. Champion stent
   P. Complete implant
   P. coronary stent
   P. laser
   P. nitinol stent
   P. pacemaker

Paramax cruciate guide system

Parasmillie double-bladed
   knife

Parham
   P. band
   P.-Martin band
   P.-Martin bone-holding
     clamp
   P.-Martin fracture
     apparatus

Parker
   P. clamp
   P. double-ended retractor
   P. fixation forceps
   P. needle
   P. tenotomy knife
   P. thumb retractor
   P. tube

Parker (*continued*)
P.-Kerr basting suture
P.-Kerr forceps
P.-Kerr intestinal clamp

P.A.S. Port catheter

Passager
P. device
P. endoprosthesis
P. introducing sheath
P. stent

Passport Balloon-on-a-Wire
dilatation catheter

Passy-Muir tracheostomy
speaking valve

paste
Osteofil allograft p.
Regenafil allograft p.
Replicare p.
Unna p.

patch
BioGlue surgical p.
Cardiofix Pericardium p.
Carrel p.
Dacron intracardiac p.
Donaldson eye p.
Fluoropassiv thin-wall
carotid p.
FTO eye p.
Hemarrest p.
Ionescu-Shiley pericardia p.
Permacol p.
polytef soft-tissue p.
Prolene Hernia system
onlay p.
RapiSeal p.
Rutkow sutureless plug and
p.
Tanne corneal p.
Testoderm p.
Tissue-Guard bovine
pericardial p.
Vascu-Guard peripheral
vascular p.
wicking glue p.

Pathfinder
P. catheter
P. exchange guidewire
P. irrigation device
P. microcatheter system
P. mini microcatheter
P. wire

peak
P. anterior compression
plate system
P. channeled plate system

Péan
P. arterial forceps
P. hemostatic clamp
P. hysterectomy clamp
P. intestinal clamp
P. scissors
P. sponge forceps
P. vessel clamp

peanut
p. dissector
p. eye implant
p. Secto dissector
p. sponge
p. sponge-holding forceps

Pearce
P. coaxial I&A cannula
P. eye speculum
P. intraocular glide
P. nucleus hydrodissector
P. Tripod cataract lens
P. vaulted-Y lens implant

Penfield
P. biopsy needle
P. dissector
P. retractor
P. silver clip
P. watchmaker suture
forceps

Pennig
P. dynamic wrist fixator
P. minifixator

Pennington
P. clamp

Pennington (*continued*)
P. hemorrhoidal forceps
P. rectal speculum
P. septal dissector
P. tissue forceps

Pentax
P. choledochocystonephro-
fiberscope
P. EUP-EC series ultrasound
gastroscope
P. FG-36UX
echoendoscope
P. fiberscope
P. flexible sigmoidoscope
P. lithotripter
P. prototype needle

Perclose closure device

pessary
Albert-Smith p.
blue ring p.
Chamber doughnut p.
Dumas p.
Gehrung p.
Gold p.
Hodge p.
Maydl p.
Mayer p.
Menge p.
Milex p.
Prentif p.
red p.
Smith retroversion p.
Vimule p.
Wylie stem p.
Zwanck radium p.

Peyman
P. intraocular forceps
P. vitrector
P. vitreous-grasping
forceps
P. wide-field lens

Phaco-Emulsifier
Cavitron P..-E.
Kelman P.-E.
MVS P.-E.

Photon
P. LaserPhaco probe
P. micro DR/VR implantable
cardioverter defibrillator

Phylax AV dual chamber
implantable cardioverter
defibrillator

Physio-Stim Lite bone-growth
stimulator

Picotip steroid-eluting lead

Pilling Weck Y-stent forceps

Pilot suturing guide

pin
Ace p.
Apex p.
Arthrex zebra p.
ARUM Colles fixation p.
ASIF screw p.
Asnis p.
Austin Moore p.
Böhler p.
Böhler-Knowles hip p.
Böhler-Steinmann p.
Barr p.
beaded hip p.
Beath p.
Belos compression p.
bevel-point Rush p.
Biofix system p.
biphasic p.
Bohlman p.
breakaway p.
Breck p.
calibrated p.
Canakis beaded hip p.
cancellous p.
Caspar distraction p.
Charnley p.
p. chuck
cloverleaf p.
Co-Cr-Mo p.
Compere threaded p.
Conley p.
cortical p.
Craig p.

pin (*continued*)
 p. crimper
 Crowe pilot point on
  Steinmann p.
 Crowe-tip p.
 Crutchfield skull-tip p.
 Davis p.
 Delitala T-p.
 deluxe FIN p.
 Denham p.
 derotational p.
 Deyerle p.
 distraction p.
 distractor p.
 duodenal p.
 Ender p.
 endodontic p.
 Fahey p.
 Fahey-Compere p.
 femoral guide p.
 Fisher half p.
 fixation p.
 friction lock p.
 Furness-Clute p.
 Getz root canal p.
 Gingrass-Messer p.
 Gouffon hip p.
 p. guard
 p. guide
 Hagie p.
 Hahnenkratt root canal p.
 Hansen-Street p.
 Hatcher p.
 Haynes p.
 p. headholder
 p. headrest
 Hegge p.
 Hessel-Nystrom p.
 Hewson breakaway p.
 hexhead p.
 Hoffmann apex fixation p.
 Hoffmann transfixion p.
 p. holder
 hook-end intramedullary p.
 p. implant
 Intraflex intramedullary p.
 intramedullary p.
 Jones p.

pin (*continued*)
 Jurgan p.
 Küntscher femur guide p.
 Kirschner wire p.
 Knowles hip p.
 Kronendonk p.
 Kronfeld p.
 lateral guide p.
 LIH hook p.
 Link-Plus retention p.
 Lottes p.
 Marble bone p.
 Markley retention p.
 Mayfield disposable skull p.
 Mayfield skull clamp p.
 McBride p.
 mechanic's p.
 medullary p.
 metal p.
 Modny p.
 Moore fixation p.
 Moule screw p.
 Mt. Sinai skull clamp p.
 Neufeld p.
 Norman tibial p.
 Oris p.
 Ormco p.
 Orthofix p.
 orthopedic p.
 OrthoSorb absorbable p.
 osseous p.
 osteotomy p.
 partially-threaded p.
 percutaneous p.
 Pidcock p.
 pin ball system
 Pischel p.
 Pugh hip p.
 rasp p.
 resorbable polydioxanone
  p.
 restorative p.
 ReUnite orthopedic p.
 revolving Ge-68 p.
 Rhinelander p.
 Rica wire guide p.
 Riordan p.
 Rissler p.

pin (*continued*)
>   Rissler-Stille p.
>   Roger Anderson p.
>   Rush intramedullary
>   fixation p.
>   safety p.
>   Safir p.
>   Sage p.
>   Scand p.
>   Schanz p.
>   Schneider self-broaching p.
>   Schweitzer p.
>   self-broaching p.
>   self-tapering p.
>   Shantz p.
>   Shriners Hospital p.
>   skeletal p.
>   Smillie p.
>   Smith-Petersen fracture p.
>   SMo Moore p.
>   smooth p.
>   Snap fixation p.
>   spring p.
>   sprue p.
>   stabilizing guide p.
>   Stader p.
>   Steinmann calibrated p.
>   Steinmann fixation p.
>   Street p.
>   strut-type p.
>   Surgin hemorrhage
>   occluder p.
>   p. suture
>   Synthes guide p.
>   tapered p.
>   threaded guide p.
>   tibial guide p.
>   titanium half p.
>   torlone fixation p.
>   trochanteric p.
>   Turner p.
>   tutoFix cortical p.
>   union broach retention p.
>   Venable-Stuck fracture p.
>   p. vise
>   von Saal medullary p.
>   Walker hollow quill p.
>   Watanabe p.

pin (*continued*)
>   Watson-Jones guide p.
>   Webb p.
>   pin wheel
>   Zimfoam p.
>   Zimmer p.

Pitié-Salpttrière saphenous vein
  hook

Pivotal instruments

Pixie minilaparoscope

plasma
>   p. clot diffusion chamber
>   p. scalpel
>   p. TFE vascular graft

Pleatman sac

Pleur-evac
>   P. autotransfusion
>   system
>   P. chest catheter
>   P. suction tube

Pleurx pleural catheter

plug
>   Alcock p.
>   Avina female urethral p.
>   Biomet p.
>   Buck p.
>   Concept bone tunnel p.
>   Dohlman p.
>   Freeman punctum p.
>   Herniamesh surgical p.
>   Isberg scleral p.
>   Kirschner femoral
>   canal p.
>   PerFix hernia p.
>   Shiley decannulation p.
>   TearSaver punctum p.

Polaris
>   P. cage
>   P. laparoscope
>   P. reusable dissector
>   P. reusable forceps

Polar-Mate bipolar
  microcoagulator

Polarus
    P. humeral rod
    P. Plus humeral fixation
        system

Pollock atraumatic grasper

Ponsky
    P. Endo Sock retrieval bag
    P. PEG tube

Pope
    P. halo dressing
    P. Oto-Wick
    P. rectal knife
    P. wick

port
    Celsite brachial p.
    Dialock access p.
    Gill-Welsh guillotine p.
    Hassan-type p.
    Hasson blunt p.
    Infuse-A-Port p.
    OmegaPort access p.
    Thora-Port p.
    Vasport access p.
    Visiport p.
    Vortex Clear-Flow p.

Porterfield catheter

Precision
    P. Tack transvaginal anchor
        system
    P. Twist transvaginal
        anchor system

probe
    Acolysis coronary p.
    Frigitronics p.
    Somnus p.

Proceed hemostatic surgical
    sealant

Pro-Clude transparent wound
    dressing

proctoscope
    ACMI p.
    Boehm p.
    Lieberman p.

proctoscope (*continued*)
    Newman p.
    Pruitt p.
    Tuttle p.
    Welch Allyn p.
    Yeoman p.

Prolene
    P. Hernia system
    P. Hernia system connector
    P. Hernia system onlay
        patch
    P. Hernia system underlay
        patch
    P. mesh
    P. mesh sheet
    P. mesh silo
    P. polypropylene suture
    P. stitch

PROloop electrosurgical device

ProOsteon
    P. implant graft material
    P. synthetic bone implant

ProPlast
    P. graft
    P. prosthesis

Prostalac hip prosthesis

prosthesis
    Accolade hip p.
    Acticon neosphincter
    AcuMatch M series modular
        femoral hip p.
    Airprene hinged knee
    Apollo hip
    Apollo knee
    Atkinson endoprosthesis
    Becker tissue expander
    Buechel-Pappas total ankle
        p.
    Caffiniere p.
    Calnan-Nicolle synthetic
        joint p.
    Carbo-Seal ascending aortic
        p.
    CardioFix pericardium
        patch

prosthesis (*continued*)
   Deon hip
   Dilamezinsert penile
   DoubleStent biliary
    endoprosthesis
   Dynaflex penile
   Finn hinged knee
    replacement
   Freestyle aortic root
    bioprosthesis
   Gianturco expandable
    metallic biliary stent
   Guepar II hinged knee
   Hanger ComfortFlex knee
   IntraStent DoubleStrut
    biliary endoprosthesis
   Judet hip
   Lord total hip
   Metasul metal-on-metal hip
   Noiles posterior stabilized
    knee
   Noiles rotating hinge total
    knee
   Omnifit HA Hip stem
   Panje voice button
    laryngeal
   Passy-Muir tracheostomy
    speaking valve
   PCA knee
   Perfecta hip
   Pillet hand
   piston stapes
   Pitt talking tracheostomy
    tube
   Prostalac hip p.
   Protek joint
   Provox speaking valve
   Ring hip
   St. George total elbow

prosthesis (*continued*)
   Wallstent iliac
    endoprosthesis
   Wehrs incus

Protector meniscus suturing
 system

Proximate
   P. disposable skin stapler
   P. flexible linear stapler
   P. linear cutter

pump
   Acat 1 intra-aortic balloon
    p.
   AutoCat intra-aortic balloon
    p.
   Hardy-Sella p.
   Reitan CatheterPump

punch
   Abrahms pleural biopsy p.
   Acufex rotary p.
   Stammberger antrum p.
   Tanne corneal p.

Punctur-Guard
   P.-G. Revolution safety
    needle holder
   P.-G. Winged Set

Pursuer helical or mini-helical
 stone basket

Putti
   P. arthroplasty gouge
   P. bone file
   P. bone rasp
   P. frame
   P. splint

Pylon intramedulary nail system

Q

Quadripolar cutting forceps

Questus
- Q. Leading Edge grasper cutter
- Q. sheathed knife

QuickDop probe

QuickDraw venous cannula

QuickSilver guide wire

Quinton
- Q. Mahurkar dual lumen cathetre
- Q. PermaCath
- Q. suction biopsy instrument
- Q. tube

Quinton-Schribner shunt

Quixil fibrin sealant

QwikStrip adhesive bandage

R

Radial Jaw single-use biopsy
  forceps

Radiofocus Glidewire

RAE endotracheal tube

Ramirez shunt

Ranawat/Burstein total hip
  system

Rancho
  R. cube
  R. fixation system
  R. Los Amigos splint
  R. swivel hinge

Rand microballoon

Raney clip

Ranfac
  R. cannula
  R. cholangiographic
    catheter
  R. KPL laparoscopic knot
    pusher
  R. soft-tissue needle

RAP cannula

Rapide suture

Rapidflap

Rapidgraft arterial vessel
  substitute

RapiSeal patch

Rashkind
  R. cardiac device
  R double umbrella device

rasp
  Aagesen disposable r.
  FeatherTouch automated r.

Raulerson syringe

Ray TFC threaded fusion cage

Raz double-prong ligature
  carrier

Razi cannula introducer

RazorVac ArthroWand

Rebar microcatheter

Reddick
  R. cystic duct
    cholangiogram catheter

Reddick-Saye suture grasper

Redifurl TaperSeal IAB catheter

Reese
  R. dermatome
  R. stimulator

Reflex anterior cervical plate
  system

ReFlex wand

Ref-Star EP catheter

Relay cardiac pacemaker

Reliance urinary control insert

Rely balloon catheter

Re-New laparoscopic
  instruments

Repela surgical glove

resector
  Linvatec Lightning blade r.
  Tiger blade r.
  UltraCut blade r.
  Mainz pouch urinary r.

Resolve Quickanchor

Response catheter

Res-Q Micron implantable
  cardioverter-defibrillator

Restore
  R. ACL guide system
  R. alginate wound dressing
  R. orthobiologic soft-tissue
    implant

retractor

retractor (*continued*)
- Abadie self-retaining r.
- Ablaza aortic wall r.
- Ablaza-Blanco cardiac valve r.
- Abramson r.
- Adams r.
- Adamson r.
- Adson brain r.
- Adson cerebellar r.
- Adson splanchnic r.
- Adson-Beckman r.
- Agrikola lacrimal sac r.
- airgun r.
- Airlift balloon r.
- alar r.
- Alden r.
- Alexander r.
- Alexander-Ballen orbital r.
- Alexander-Matson r.
- Alexian Hospital r.
- Alfreck r.
- Allen r.
- Allis lung r.
- Allison lung r.
- Allport mastoid bayonet r.
- Allport-Babcock r.
- Allport-Gifford r.
- Alm microsurgery r.
- Alm self-retaining r.
- Alter lip r.
- Amenabar iris r.
- American Heyer-Schulte brain r.
- Amoils iris r.
- Anderson double-end r.
- Anderson-Adson self-retaining r.
- Andrews tracheal r.
- angled iris r.
- angled vein r.
- Ankeney sternal r.
- Ann Arbor phrenic r.
- Anthony pillar r.
- antral r.
- AOR collateral ligament r.
- aortic valve r.
- Apfelbaum cerebellar r.

retractor (*continued*)
- apicolysis r.
- appendectomy r.
- appendiceal r.
- arch rake r.
- Arem r.
- Arem-Madden r.
- arm r.
- Army-Navy r.
- Aronson esophageal r.
- Aronson lateral sternomastoid r.
- Arruga eye r.
- Arruga globe r.
- Ashley r.
- Assistant Free r.
- Aston nasal r.
- Aston submental r.
- atrial septal r.
- Aufranc cobra r.
- Aufranc femoral neck r.
- Aufranc hip r.
- Aufranc psoas r.
- Aufranc push r.
- Aufricht nasal r.
- Austin dental r.
- automatic skin r.
- Auvard weighted vaginal r.
- Azar iris r.
- Babcock r.
- baby Adson brain r.
- baby Balfour r.
- baby Collin abdominal r.
- baby Roux r.
- baby Senn-Miller r.
- baby Weitlaner self-retaining r.
- Backmann thyroid r.
- Bacon cranial r.
- Badgley laminectomy r.
- Bahnson sternal r.
- Bakelite r.
- Balfour center-blade abdominal r.
- Balfour pediatric abdominal r.
- Balfour retractor with fenestrated blade

retractor (*continued*)

Balfour self-retaining r.
ball-type r.
Ballantine
   hemilaminectomy r.
Ballen-Alexander orbital r.
Bankart rectal r.
Bankart shoulder r.
Barkan bident r.
Baron r.
Barr self-retaining rectal r.
Barraquer lid r.
Barraquer-Krumeich-
   Swinger r.
Barrett-Adson cerebellum r.
Barron r.
Barsky nasal r.
Bauer r.
Beardsley esophageal r.
Beatty pillar r.
Beaver r.
beaver-tail r.
Bechert-Kratz cannulated
   nucleus r.
Becker r.
Beckman goiter r.
Beckman self-retaining r.
Beckman thyroid r.
Beckman-Adson
   laminectomy r.
Beckman-Eaton
   laminectomy r.
Beckman-Weitlaner
   laminectomy r.
Bellfield wire r.
Bellman r.
Bellucci-Wullstein r.
Benedict r.
Beneventi self-retaining r.
Bennett bone r.
Bennett tibial r.
bent malleable r.
Berens esophageal r.
Berens lid r.
Berens mastectomy skin
   flap r.
Berens thyroid r.
Bergen r.

retractor (*continued*)

Bergman tracheal r.
Bergman wound r.
Berkeley r.
Berkeley-Bonney self-
   retaining abdominal r.
Berlind-Auvard r.
Berna infant abdominal r.
Bernay tracheal r.
Bernstein nasal r.
Bertin hip r.
Bethune phrenic r.
Bicek vaginal r.
bident r.
Biestek thyroid r.
bifid gallbladder r.
bifurcated r.
Biggs mammoplasty r.
biliary r.
Billroth ovarian r.
Billroth-Stille r.
Bishop r.
bivalved r.
Black r.
bladder r.
Blair four-prong r.
Blair-Brown vacuum r.
Blakesley uvular r.
Blanco r.
Bland perineal r.
Blount double-prong r.
Blount hip r.
Blount knee r.
Blount single-prong r.
blunt rake r.
boardlike r.
Bodnar knee r.
Boley r.
bone r.
Bookwalter ring r.
Bookwalter-Balfour r.
Bookwalter-Goulet r.
Bookwalter-Harrington r.
Bookwalter-Hill-Ferguson
   rectal r.
Bookwalter-Kelly r.
Bookwalter-Magrina vaginal
   r.

retractor (*continued*)
- Bookwalter-St. Mark deep pelvic r.
- Bose r.
- Bosworth nerve root r.
- bowel r.
- Boyd r.
- Boyes-Goodfellow hook r.
- Braastad costal arch r.
- brain silicone-coated r.
- Brantley-Turner vaginal r.
- Brawley scleral wound r.
- Breen r.
- Breisky vaginal r.
- Breisky-Navratil straight r.
- Brewster phrenic r.
- Briggs r.
- Brinker hygienic tissue r.
- Bristow-Bankart humeral r.
- Bristow-Bankart soft tissue r.
- Brompton Hospital r.
- Bronson-Turtz iris r.
- Brophy tenaculum r.
- Brown uvular r.
- Brown-Burr modified Gillies r.
- Bruch mastoid r.
- Bruening r.
- Brunner r.
- Brunschwig visceral r.
- Bucy spinal cord r.
- Budde halo neurosurgical r.
- Budde halo ring r.
- Buie r.
- Buie-Smith anal r.
- bulb r.
- Bulnes-Sanchez r.
- Burford rib r.
- Burford-Finochietto rib r.
- Busenkell posterior hip r.
- Butler dental r.
- Butler pillar r.
- buttonhook nerve r.
- Bycroft-Brunswick thyroid r.
- Byford r.
- Cairns scalp r.
- Callahan r.

retractor (*continued*)
- Campbell lacrimal sac r.
- Campbell nerve root r.
- Campbell self-retaining r.
- Campbell suprapubic r.
- Canadian chest r.
- Cardillo r.
- cardiovascular r.
- Carlens tracheotomy r.
- Carlens-Stille tracheal r.
- Caroline finger r.
- Carroll offset hand r.
- Carroll self-retaining spring r.
- Carroll-Bennett finger r.
- Carten mitral valve r.
- Carter r.
- Caspar cervical r.
- Castallo eyelid r.
- Castaneda infant sternal r.
- Castroviejo adjustable r.
- Castroviejo lid r.
- cat's paw r.
- Cave knee r.
- cecostomy r.
- Cer-View lateral vaginal r.
- cerebellar r.
- cerebral r.
- cervical disk r.
- chalazion r.
- Chamberlain-Fries atraumatic r.
- Chandler knee r.
- Chandler laminectomy r.
- channel r.
- Charnley horizontal r.
- Charnley initial incision r.
- Charnley knee r.
- Charnley pin r.
- Charnley self-retaining r.
- Charnley standard stem r.
- Cheanvechai-Favaloro r.
- cheek r.
- Cherry laminectomy self-retaining r.
- Cherry S-shaped brain r.
- Cheyne r.
- Children's Hospital pediatric r.

retractor (*continued*)
    Chitten-Hill r.
    Christie gallbladder r.
    Cibis-Vaiser muscle r.
    claw r.
    Clayman lid r.
    Clevedent r.
    Cleveland IMA r.
    r. clip
    Cloward blade r.
    Cloward brain r.
    Cloward cervical r.
    Cloward dural r.
    Cloward nerve root r.
    Cloward self-retaining r.
    Cloward tissue r.
    Cloward-Cushing vein r.
    Cloward-Hoen
        laminectomy r.
    Cobb r.
    cobra-head r.
    Cocke large flap r.
    Cohen r.
    Cole duodenal r.
    Coleman r.
    collapsible tissue r.
    collar-button iris r.
    Collin abdominal r.
    Collin sternal self-retaining
        r.
    Collin-Hartmann r.
    Collins-Mayo mastoid r.
    Collis anterior cervical r.
    Collis posterior lumbar r.
    Collis-Taylor r.
    Colonial r.
    Colver tonsillar r.
    Comyns-Berkeley r.
    condylar neck r.
    Cone laminectomy r.
    Cone scalp r.
    Cone self-retaining r.
    contour scalp r.
    Converse blade r.
    Converse double-ended
        alar r.
    Converse nasal r.
    Conway lid r.

retractor (*continued*)
    Cook rectal r.
    Cooley aortic r.
    Cooley atrial valve r.
    Cooley carotid r.
    Cooley femoral r.
    Cooley mitral valve r.
    Cooley MPC cardiovascular
        r.
    Cooley neonatal sternal r.
    Cooley rib r.
    Cooley sternotomy r.
    Cooley-Merz sternal r.
    Cooley-Merz sternum r.
    Cope double-ended r.
    corner r.
    corrugated forehead r.
    cortex r.
    Coryllos r.
    Cosgrove mitral valve r.
    costal arch r.
    Costenbader r.
    Coston-Trent iris r.
    Cottle alar r.
    Cottle four-prong r.
    Cottle hook r.
    Cottle nasal r.
    Cottle pillar r.
    Cottle pronged r.
    Cottle sharp-prong r.
    Cottle single-blade r.
    Cottle soft palate r.
    Cottle upper lateral
        exposing r.
    Cottle weighted r.
    Cottle-Joseph r.
    Cottle-Neivert r.
    Crafoord r.
    Craig-Sheehan r.
    cranial r.
    crank frame r.
    Crawford aortic r.
    Crego periosteal r.
    Crile thyroid double-ended
        r.
    Crockard hard palate r.
    Crockard pharyngeal r.
    Crotti goiter r.

retractor (*continued*)

    Crotti thyroid r.
    Crowe-Davis mouth r.
    Cushing aluminum r.
    Cushing angled
      decompression r.
    Cushing bivalve r.
    Cushing brain r.
    Cushing decompression r.
    Cushing nerve r.
    Cushing S-shaped r.
    Cushing self-retaining r.
    Cushing straight r.
    Cushing subtemporal r.
    Cushing vein r.
    Cushing-Kocher r.
    dacryocystorhinostomy r.
    Dallas r.
    Danek self-retaining r.
    Danis r.
    Darling popliteal r.
    Darrach r.
    Dautrey r.
    David-Baker eyelid r.
    Davidoff trigeminal r.
    Davidson erector spinae r.
    Davidson scapular r.
    Davis brain r.
    Davis double-ended r.
    Davis pillar r.
    Davis self-retaininig scalp r.
    de la Plaza
      transconjunctival r.
    Deaver pediatric r.
    DeBakey chest r.
    DeBakey-Balfour r.
    DeBakey-Cooley Deaver-
      type r.
    Decker r.
    decompressive r.
    Dedo laser r.
    deep abdominal r.
    deep blunt rake r.
    deep Deaver r.
    DeLaginiere abdominal r.
    Delaney phrenic r.
    DeLee corner r.
    DeLee Universal r.

retractor (*continued*)

    DeLee vaginal r.
    DeLee vesical r.
    DeMartel self-retaining
      brain r.
    Denis Browne pediatric r.
    Denis Browne ring r.
    dental r.
    Denver-Wells atrial r.
    Denver-Wells sternal r.
    DePuy r.
    D'Errico nerve root r.
    D'Errico-Adson r.
    Desmarres cardiovascular r.
    Desmarres lid r.
    Desmarres valve r.
    Desmarres vein r.
    Deucher abdominal r.
    Devine-Millard-Aufricht r.
    Di-Main r.
    Dingman flexible r.
    Dingman Flexsteel r.
    Dingman zygoma hook r.
    Dingman-Senn r.
    disposable iris r.
    Dixon center-blade r.
    Doane knee r.
    Dockhorn r.
    dog chain r.
    Dohn-Carton brain r.
    Dorsey nerve root r.
    Dorton self-retaining r.
    Dott r.
    double-bent Hohmann
      acetabular r.
    double-cobra r.
    double-crank r.
    double-ended r.
    double-fishhook r.
    Downing II laminectomy r.
    Doyen child abdominal r.
    Doyen vaginal r.
    Dozier radiolucent Bennett
      r.
    Drews iris r.
    Drews-Rosenbaum iris r.
    dual nerve root suction r.
    Duane r.

retractor (*continued*)
dull r.
dull-pronged r.
Dumont r.
duodenal r.
dural suction r.
Duryea r.
East-West soft tissue r.
Eastman vaginal r.
Eccentric "Y" adjustable
finger r.
Echols r.
Eddey parotid r.
Edinburgh brain r.
Effenberger r.
Elias lid r.
Eliasoph lid r.
Elite Farley r.
Elschnig lid r.
Emmet obstetrical r.
Emory EndoPlastic r.
endaural r.
Endoflex endoscopic r.
EndoRetract r.
Endotrac r.
Enker self-retaining
brain r.
epicardial r.
epiglottis r.
erector spinae r.
ESI long, narrow
mammoplasty r.
esophageal r.
examination r.
eXpose r.
externofrontal r.
extraoral sigmoid notch r.
eyelid r.
facelift r.
Falk vaginal r.
fan elevator r.
fan liver r.
Farabeuf double-ended r.
Farley Elite spinal r.
Farmingdale r.
Farr self-retaining r.
Farr spring r.
Farr wire r.

retractor (*continued*)
Fasanella double-ended iris
r.
fat pad r.
Favaloro atrial r.
Favaloro self-retaining
sternal r.
Federspiel cheek r.
Feldman lid r.
femoral neck r.
Ferguson r.
Ferguson-Moon rectal r.
Fernstroem bladder r.
Fernstroem-Stille r.
Ferris Smith orbital r.
Ferris Smith-Sewall orbital
r.
fiberoptic r.
finger rake r.
Fink lacrimal r.
Finochietto hand r.
Finochietto infant rib r.
Finochietto laminectomy r.
Finochietto-Geissendorfer
rib r.
Finsen r.
Fisch dural r.
Fisher double-ended r.
Fisher fenestrated lid r.
Fisher lid r.
Fisher tonsillar r.
Fisher-Nugent r.
five-prong rake blade r.
fixed ring r.
flexible translimbal iris r.
FlexPosure endoscopic r.
Flexsteel ribbon r.
Foerster abdominal r.
Fomon hook r.
Fomon nasal r.
force fulcrum r.
Ford-Deaver r.
Forker r.
Foss bifid gallbladder r.
Foss biliary r.
four-prong r.
Fowler self-retaining r.
Franklin malleable r.

retractor (*continued*)
    Franz abdominal r.
    Frater intracardiac r.
    Frazier cerebral r.
    Frazier laminectomy r.
    Frazier lighted r.
    Frazier-Fay r.
    Freeman facelift r.
    Freer dural r.
    Freer skin r.
    Freer submucous r.
    Freiberg hip r.
    Freiberg nerve root r.
    Freidrich-Ferguson r.
    French S-shaped brain r.
    French-Stern-McCarthy r.
    Friedman perineal r.
    Friedman vaginal r.
    Fritsch abdominal r.
    Fujita snake r.
    Fukuda humeral head r.
    Fukushima r.
    Fullerview flexible iris r.
    Fulton r.
    Gabarro r.
    gallbladder r.
    gallows-type r.
    Gam-Mer medial
        esophageal r.
    Gam-Mer occipital r.
    Gant gallbladder r.
    Garrett peripheral vascular r.
    Garrigue vaginal r.
    gastric resection r.
    Gaubatz rib r.
    Gauthier r.
    Gazayerli endoscopic r.
    Gazayerli-Mediflex r.
    Geissendorfer rib r.
    Gelpi abdominal r.
    Gelpi perineal r.
    Gelpi self-retaining r.
    Gelpi vaginal r.
    Gelpi-Lowrie r.
    general r.
    Gerbode sternal r.
    Gerow-Harrington heart-
        shaped distal end r.

retractor (*continued*)
    Ghazi rib r.
    Gibson-Balfour abdominal r.
    Gifford mastoid r.
    Gifford scalp r.
    Gifford-Jansen mastoid r.
    Gil-Vernet lumbotomy r.
    Gil-Vernet renal sinus r.
    Gillies single-hook skin r.
    Givner lid r.
    Glaser laminectomy r.
    Glass abdominal r.
    Glenner vaginal r.
    Goelet double-ended r.
    goiter r.
    Goldstein lacrimal sac r.
    Goligher modification of the
        Berkeley-Bonney r.
    Goligher sternal-lifting r.
    Gomez gastric r.
    Gooch mastoid r.
    Good r.
    Goodhill r.
    Goodyear tonsillar r.
    Gosset abdominal r.
    Gosset appendectomy r.
    Gosset self-retaininig r.
    Gott malleable r.
    Gradle eyelid r.
    Graether r.
    Grant gallbladder r.
    Gray surgical r.
    Green goiter r.
    Green thyroid r.
    Greenberg Universal r.
    Greenberg-Sugita r.
    Greenwald r.
    Grice r.
    Grieshaber flexible iris r.
    Grieshaber self-retaining r.
    Grieshaber spring wire r.
    Grieshaber-Balfour r.
    Groenholm lid r.
    Gross iris r.
    Gross patent ductus r.
    Gross-Pomeranz-Watkins
        atrial r.
    Gross-Pomeranz-Watkins r.

retractor (*continued*)

Gruenwald r.
Guilford-Wright meatal r.
Guthrie r.
Guttmann obstetrical r.
Guttmann vaginal r.
Guzman-Blanco
  epiglottic r.
Haight pulmonary r.
Haight rib r.
Haight-Finochietto rib r.
Hajek antral r.
Hajek lip r.
half-moon r.
halo r.
Hamburger-Brennan-
  Mahorner thyroid r.
Hamby brain r.
Hamby-Hibbs r.
hand r.
hand-held r.
hard palate r.
Hardy lip r.
Hardy-Duddy vaginal r.
Harken rib r.
Harrington bladder r.
Harrington Britetrac r.
Harrington splanchnic r.
Harrington sympathectomy
  r.
Harrington-Deaver r.
Harrington-Pemberton
  sympathectomy r.
Harrison chalazion r.
Hartstein irrigating iris r.
Hartzler rib r.
Haslinger palate r.
Haslinger uvular r.
Hasson r.
Haverfield
  hemilaminectomy r.
Haverfield-Scoville
  hemilaminectomy r.
Haynes r.
Hays finger r.
Hays hand r.
Heaney hysterectomy r.
Heaney vaginal r.

retractor (*continued*)

Heaney-Simon
  hysterectomy r.
Heaney-Simon vaginal r.
Hedblom rib r.
Heifitz r.
Heiss mastoid r.
Heiss soft tissue r.
Helfrick anal r.
Helveston "Great Big
  Barbie" r.
hemilaminectomy r.
Henderson self-retaining r.
Henley carotid r.
Henner endaural r.
Henner T-model endaural r.
Henning meniscal r.
Henrotin r.
hernia r.
Hertzler baby rib r.
Hess nerve root r.
Heyer-Schulte brain r.
Hibbs self-retaining
  laminectomy r.
Hill rectal r.
Hill-Ferguson rectal r.
Hillis eyelid r.
Himmelstein sternal r.
Hirschman r.
Hoen hemilaminectomy r.
Hoen scalp r.
Hohmann r.
Holman lung r.
Holscher nerve r.
Holzbach abdominal r.
Holzheimer mastoid r.
Holzheimer skin r.
Homan r.
hook r.
r. hook
Horgan r.
horizontal flexible bar r.
Hosel r.
House hand-held double-
  end r.
House-Urban middle fossa
  r.
Howorth toothed r.

retractor (*continued*)
   Huang Universal arm r.
   Hubbard r.
   Hudson bone r.
   humeral r.
   Hunt bladder r.
   Hupp tracheal r.
   Hurd tonsillar pillar r.
   Hurson flexible r.
   Hutchinson iris r.
   hysterectomy r.
   IMA r.
   incision r.
   infant abdominal r.
   infant eyelid r.
   infant rib r.
   Inge laminectomy r.
   initial incision r.
   intestinal occlusion r.
   intracardiac r.
   intradural r.
   iris r.
   Iron Intern r.
   irrigating mushroom r.
   Israel blunt rake r.
   Jackson self-retaining
      goiter r.
   Jackson tracheal r.
   Jackson vaginal r.
   Jacobson bladder r.
   Jacobson goiter r.
   Jaeger lid r.
   Jaffe wire lid r.
   Jaffe-Givner lid r.
   Jako laser r.
   Jannetta posterior fossa r.
   Jansen mastoid r.
   Jansen scalp r.
   Jansen-Gifford mastoid r.
   Jansen-Wagner
      mastoid r.
   Jarit cross-action r.
   Jarit P.E.E.R. r.
   Jarit renal sinus r.
   Jarit spring-wire r.
   Jarit-Deaver r.
   Jefferson self-retaining r.
   Joe's hoe r.

retractor (*continued*)
   Johns Hopkins gallbladder r.
   Johnson cheek r.
   Johnson hook r.
   Johnson ventriculogram r.
   Jones IMA epicardial r.
   Jorgenson r.
   Joseph skin hook r.
   Joseph wound r.
   Joystick r.
   Judd-Allis intestinal r.
   Judd-Mason bladder r.
   Judd-Mason prostatic r.
   Kalamarides dural r.
   Kanavel-Senn r.
   Kapp Surgical Instrument
      total knee r.
   Karmody vascular spring r.
   Kartush insulated r.
   Kasdan r.
   Kaufer type II r.
   Kaufman type II r.
   Keeler-Fison tissue r.
   Keeler-Rodger iris r.
   Keizer lid r.
   Keizer-Lancaster lid r.
   Kel r.
   Kelly abdominal r.
   Kelly-Sims vaginal r.
   Kelman iris r.
   Kennerdell medial orbital r.
   Kennerdell-Maroon orbital
      r.
   Kerrison r.
   kidney r.
   Killey molar r.
   Killian-King goiter r.
   Kilner nasal r.
   Kilner skin hook r.
   Kilpatrick r.
   King self-retaining goiter r.
   King-Hurd r.
   Kirby lid r.
   Kirchner r.
   Kirkland r.
   Kirklin atrial r.
   Kirschenbaum r.
   Kirschner abdominal r.

retractor (*continued*)

Kirschner-Balfour
  abdominal r.
Kitner r.
Kleinert-Kutz hook r.
Kleinert-Ragnell r.
Kleinsasser r.
Klemme appendectomy r.
Klemme gasserian ganglion
  r.
Klemme laminectomy r.
Kliners alar r.
Knapp lacrimal sac r.
knee r.
Knighton hemilaminectomy
  self-retaining r.
Kobayashi r.
Kocher bladder r.
Kocher blade r.
Kocher bone r.
Kocher gallbladder r.
Kocher self-retaining goiter r.
Kocher-Crotti self-retaining
  goiter r.
Kocher-Langenbeck r.
Kocher-Wagner r.
Koenig vein r.
Koerte r.
Koneg r.
Korte r.
Korte-Wagner r.
Kozlinski r.
Krönlein-Berke r.
Krasky r.
Kretschmer r.
Kristeller vaginal r.
Kronfeld eyelid r.
Kuda r.
Kuglen lens r.
Kuyper-Murphy sternal r.
Kwapis subcondylar r.
Lack tongue r.
lacrimal sac r.
Lahey Clinic nerve root r.
Lahey goiter r.
Lahey thyroid r.
laminectomy self-retaining
  r.

retractor (*continued*)

Landau vaginal r.
Landon narrow-bladed r.
Lane r.
Lange bone r.
Lange-Hohmann bone r.
Langenbeck periosteal r.
Langenbeck-Cushing vein r.
Langenbeck-Green r.
Langenbeck-Mannerfelt r.
Laplace liver r.
laryngeal r.
laryngofissure r.
lateral wall r.
Latrobe soft palate r.
Lawton-Balfour
  self-retaining r.
leaflet r.
Leasure tracheal r.
Leatherman trochanteric r.
Lee double-ended r.
Legen self-retaining r.
Legueu bladder r.
Legueu kidney r.
Lemmon self-retaining
  sternal r.
Lemole atrial valve
  self-retaining r.
Lemole mitral valve r.
Lempert r.
Lempert-Colver r.
LeVasseur-Merrill r.
Levinthal surgery r.
Levy articulating r.
Levy perineal r.
Lewis r.
Leyla self-retaining brain r.
Leyla-Yasargil self-retaining
  r.
lid r.
Liddicoat aortic valve r.
lighted r.
LightWare micro r.
Lilienthal-Sauerbruch r.
Lillehei r.
Lillie r.
Linton splanchnic r.
lip r.

retractor (*continued*)
  Little r.
  liver r.
  Lockhart-Mummery r.
  Lofberg thyroid r.
  Logan lacrimal sac self-retaining r.
  London narrow-bladed r.
  Lone Star r.
  long atraumatic r.
  loop r.
  Lorie cheek r.
  Lothrop tonsillar r.
  Lothrop uvular r.
  Love nasopharyngeal r.
  Love nerve root r.
  Love uvula r.
  Lovejoy r.
  Lowman hand r.
  Lowsley prostate r.
  Luer double-ended tracheal r.
  Luer S-shaped r.
  Lukens double-ended tracheal r.
  Lukens epiglottic r.
  Lukens thymus r.
  lumbar r.
  lumbotomy r.
  lung r.
  Luongo hand r.
  Luther-Peter r.
  MacAusland muscle r.
  MacAusland-Kelly r.
  McBurney fenestrated r.
  McBurney thyroid r.
  McCabe antral r.
  McCabe parotidectomy r.
  McCabe posterior fossa r.
  McCool capsule r.
  McCullough externofrontal r.
  McGannon iris r.
  McGill r.
  McIndoe r.
  MacKay contour self-retaining r.
  MacKool capsule r.

retractor (*continued*)
  McNealey visceral r.
  MacVicar double-end strabismus r.
  Magrina-Bookwalter vaginal r.
  Mahorner thyroid r.
  Maison r.
  Maliniac nasal r.
  Malis cerebellar r.
  Malis cerebral r.
  malleable blade r.
  malleable copper r.
  malleable ribbon r.
  malleable stainless steel r.
  Maltz r.
  mandibular body r.
  Mannerfelt r.
  Manning r.
  manual r.
  Mark II "S" total knee r.
  Mark II "Z" knee r.
  Mark II Chandler total knee r.
  Mark II concave total knee r.
  Mark II lateral collateral ligament r.
  Mark II modular weighted r.
  Mark II PCL r.
  Mark II Stubbs short-prong collateral ligament r.
  Mark II wide PCL knee r.
  Markham-Meyerding hemilaminectomy r.
  Markley r.
  Martin abdominal r.
  Martin cheek r.
  Martin lip r.
  Martin nerve root r.
  Martin palate r.
  Martin rectal hook r.
  Martin vaginal r.
  Mason-Judd bladder r.
  Mason-Judd self-retaining r.
  mastectomy skin flap r.
  mastoid self-retaining r.
  Mathieu double-ended r.

retractor (*continued*)

Matson-Mead apicolysis r.
Mattison-Upshaw r.
Mayfield r.
Mayo abdominal r.
Mayo-Adams
  appendectomy r.
Mayo-Adams self-retaining
  r.
Mayo-Collins
  appendectomy r.
Mayo-Collins double-ended
  r.
Mayo-Collins mastoid r.
Mayo-Lovelace abdominal
  r.
Mayo-Simpson r.
meat hook r.
Medicon rib r.
Mediflex Gazayerli r.
Meigs r.
Meller lacrimal sac r.
meniscal r.
Merrill-Levassier r.
metacarpal double-
  ended r.
metal bar r.
Meyer biliary r.
Meyerding finger r.
Meyerding self-retaining
  laminectomy r.
Meyerding-Deaver r.
microlumbar diskectomy r.
microsurgical r.
microvascular modified
  Alm r.
middle fossa r.
Middledorf r.
Middlesex-Pointe r.
Mikulicz abdominal r.
Mikulicz liver r.
Miles r.
Milex r.
Miller r.
Miller-Senn double-ended r.
Milligan self-retaining r.
Millin retropublic bladder r.
Millin self-retaining r.

retractor (*continued*)

Millin-Bacon bladder
  self-retaining r.
Millin-Bacon retropubic
  prostatectomy r.
Miltex r.
mini-Hohmann r.
Minnesota r.
Miskimon cerebellar
  self-retaining r.
mitral valve r.
Moberg r.
Moberg-Stille r.
Mollison self-retaining r.
Moon rectal r.
Moore bone r.
Moorehead cheek r.
Moorehead dental r.
Morris r.
Morrison-Hurd pillar r.
Morse modified Finochietto
  r.
Morse sternal r.
Morse valve r.
Mosher lifesaver r.
Mott double-ended r.
Mueller lacrimal sac r.
Mueller-Balfour
  self-retaining r.
Mufson-Cushing r.
Muldoon lid r.
multiprong rake r.
multipurpose r.
Munro self-retaining r.
Murless head r.
Murphy gallbladder r.
Murphy rake r.
Murphy-Balfour r.
Murtagh self-retaining infant
  scalp r.
Naclerio diaphragm r.
narrow Deaver r.
nasal r.
nasopharyngeal r.
Navratil r.
Neivert double-ended r.
Nelson self-retaining rib r.
neonatal sternal r.

retractor (*continued*)
    nerve root r.
    Nevyas drape r.
    New tracheal r.
    New York Hospital r.
    newborn eyelid r.
    Newell lid r.
    Newton-Morgan r.
    Noblock r.
    North-South r.
    Nuttall r.
    Nystroem r.
    Nystroem-Stille r.
    Oberhill self-retaining r.
    O'Brien phrenic r.
    O'Brien rib r.
    obstetrical r.
    Obwegeser channel r.
    Obwegeser periosteal r.
    Ochsner malleable r.
    Ochsner ribbon r.
    Ochsner vascular r.
    Ochsner-Favaloro
        self-retaining r.
    O'Connor abdominal r.
    O'Connor vaginal r.
    O'Connor-O'Sullivan
        abdominal r.
    O'Connor-O'Sullivan
        self-retaining vaginal r.
    Octopus r.
    Oertli wire lid r.
    Oettingen abdominal
        self-retaining r.
    offset hand r.
    Oklahoma iris wire r.
    Oldberg brain r.
    Oldberg straight r.
    Oliver scalp r.
    Ollier rake r.
    Omni r.
    Omni-Tract vaginal r.
    orbicular r.
    O'Reilly esophageal r.
    orbital r.
    Orley r.
    Osher iris r.
    Osher lid r.

retractor (*continued*)
    O'Sullivan self-retaining
        abdominal r.
    O'Sullivan vaginal r.
    O'Sullivan-O'Connor
        self-retaining abdominal r.
    O'Sullivan-O'Connor vaginal
        r.
    r. oval sprocket frame
    Packiam r.
    palate r.
    Paparella self-retaining r.
    Paparella-Weitlaner r.
    Parker double-ended r.
    Parker thumb r.
    Parker-Mott double-ended
        r.
    Parkes nasal r.
    Parks anal r.
    parotidectomy r.
    Parsonnet epicardial r.
    patent ductus r.
    Paul lacrimal sac r.
    Paulson knee r.
    Payne r.
    Payr abdominal r.
    Peck rake r.
    pediatric abdominal r.
    pediatric self-retaining r.
    Peet lighted splanchnic r.
    Pemberton r.
    Pemco r.
    Penfield r.
    Percy amputation r.
    Percy bone r.
    Percy-Wolfson gallbladder
        r.
    periareolar r.
    perineal prostatectomy r.
    perineal self-retaining r.
    peripheral vascular r.
    Perkins otologic r.
    Perman-Stille abdominal r.
    pharyngeal r.
    Pheifer-Young r.
    phrenic r.
    Pickrell r.
    Picot vaginal r.

retractor (*continued*)
Pierce cheek r.
pillar r.
pillar-and-post
   microsurgical r.
Pilling r.
Pilling-Favaloro r.
Piper lateral wall r.
Plester r.
Poliak eye r.
Polytrac Gomez r.
Pomeranz hiatal hernia r.
popliteal r.
Poppen-Gelpi laminectomy
   self-retaining r.
Portmann r.
Posada-Vasco orbital r.
postauricular r.
posterior fossa r.
posterior urethral r.
Pratt bivalve r.
Proctor cheek r.
pronged r.
prostatic r.
Proud-White uvula r.
Pryor-Péan vaginal r.
psoas r.
pulmonary r.
Purcell self-retaining
   abdominal r.
Quervain abdominal r.
Quervain-Sauerbruch r.
Radcliff perineal r.
Ragnell double-ended r.
Ragnell-Davis double-ended
   r.
rake r.
Ralks ear r.
Raney laminectomy r.
Rankin prostatic r.
Raylor malleable r.
rectal hook r.
Rees lighted r.
Rehbein infant abdominal r.
Rehne abdominal r.
Reinhart r.
Remine mastectomy skin
   flap r.

retractor (*continued*)
renal sinus r.
retaining r.
retractor blade
retropubic prostatectomy r.
rib r.
ribbon malleable r.
Rica brain r.
Rica mastoid r.
Rica multipurpose r.
Rica posterior cranial fossa
   r.
Rica scalp r.
Ricard abdominal r.
Richards abdominal r.
Richardson abdominal r.
Richardson appendectomy
   r.
Richardson-Eastman
   double-ended r.
Richter vaginal r.
Rigby abdominal r.
Rigby appendectomy r.
Rigby bivalve r.
Rigby rectal r.
Rigby vaginal r.
right-angle r.
ring abdominal r.
Rissler kidney r.
Rizzo r.
Rizzuti iris r.
Roberts thumb r.
Robin-Masse abdominal r.
Robinson lung r.
Rochester atrial septal r.
Rochester colonial r.
Rochester rake r.
Rochester-Ferguson
   double-ended r.
Rollet eye r.
Rollet lacrimal sac r.
Rollet lake r.
Rollet skin r.
Roos brachial plexus root r.
Rose double-ended r.
Rose tracheal r.
Rosenbaum iris r.
Rosenbaum-Drews iris r.

retractor (*continued*)

Rosenbaum-Drews plastic r.
Rosenberg full-radius blade synovial r.
Rosenberg-Sampson r.
Ross aortic valve r.
Rotalok skin r.
Rothon r.
Roux double-ended r.
Rowe boathook r.
Rowe humeral head r.
Rowe orbital floor r.
Rowe scapular neck r.
Rudolph trowel r.
Rultract internal mammary artery r.
Rumel r.
Ryecroft r.
Ryerson bone r.
S-shaped brain r.
Sachs angled vein r.
Sachs-Cushing r.
Samb r.
Sanchez-Bulnes lacrimal sac self-retaining r.
Sato lid r.
Sauerbruch r.
Sauerbruch-Zukschwerdt rib r.
Sawyer rectal r.
Sayre r.
scalp self-retaining r.
Scanlan pediatric r.
scapular r.
Schepens orbital r.
Schindler r.
Schink metatarsal r.
Schnitker scalp r.
Schoenborn r.
Scholten sternal r.
Schuknecht postauricular self-retaining r.
Schuknecht-Wullstein r.
Schultz iris r.
Schwartz laminectomy self-retaining r.
scleral wound r.

retractor (*continued*)

Scoville Britetrac r.
Scoville cervical disk self-retaining r.
Scoville hemilaminectomy self-retaining r.
Scoville laminectomy r.
Scoville nerve root r.
Scoville psoas muscle r.
Scoville self-retaining r.
Scoville-Haverfield laminectomy r.
Scoville-Richter self-retaining r.
Segond abdominal r.
Seldin dental r.
Seletz-Gelpi self-retaining r.
self-adhering lid r.
self-retaining abdominal r.
self-retaining brain r.
self-retaining ring r.
self-retaining skin r.
self-retaining spring r.
Sellor rib r.
Semb lung r.
Semb self-retaining r.
Senn double-ended r.
Senn mastoid r.
Senn self-retaining r.
Senn-Dingman double-ended r.
Senn-Green r.
Senn-Kanavel double-ended r.
Senn-Miller r.
Senturia r.
serrated r.
serrefine r.
Sewall orbital r.
Shambaugh endaural self-retaining r.
sharp-pronged r.
Shearer lip r.
Sheehan r.
Sheldon hemilaminectomy self-retaining r.
Sheldon-Gosset self-retaining r.

retractor (*continued*)

Sherwin self-retaining r.
Sherwood r.
short Heaney r.
Shriners Hospital
  interlocking r.
Shuletz-Paul rib r.
Shurly tracheal r.
sigmoid notch r.
Silverstein lateral venous
  sinus r.
Simon vaginal r.
Sims double-ended r.
Sims rectal r.
Sims vaginal r.
Sims-Kelly vaginal r.
single-blade r.
single-hook r.
single-prong broad
  acetabular r.
Sisson spring r.
Sisson-Love r.
Sistrunk band r.
Sistrunk double-ended r.
six-prong rake r.
skin flap r.
skin hook r.
skin self-retaining r.
Sloan goiter self-retaining r.
Sluder palate r.
Small rake r.
Small tissue r.
SMIC cheek r.
Smillie knee joint r.
Smith anal r.
Smith nerve root suction r.
Smith rectal self-retaining r.
Smith vaginal self-retaining
  r.
Smith-Buie anal r.
Smith-Buie self-retaining
  rectal r.
Smith-Petersen capsular r.
Smithwick r.
Snitman endaural self-
  retaining r.
Sofield r.
soft palate r.

retractor (*continued*)

soft tissue blade r.
Space-OR r.
Spacekeeper r.
spike r.
spinal cord r.
Spivey iris r.
splanchnic r.
spoon r.
spring r.
spring-loaded self-retaining
  r.
spring-wire r.
Spurling r.
St. Luke's r.
St. Mark's Hospital r.
St. Mark's lipped r.
St. Mark's pelvis r.
Stack r.
Stamey dorsal vein apical r.
stay suture r.
Steiner-Auvard vaginal r.
stereotactic r.
sternal r.
sternotomy r.
Stevens lacrimal r.
Stevens muscle hook r.
Stevenson lacrimal sac r.
Stille cheek r.
Stille heart r.
Stille-Broback knee r.
Stiwer r.
Stookey r.
Storer thoracoabdominal r.
Storz r.
straight r.
Strandell r.
Strandell-Stille r.
Strully nerve root r.
Stuck self-retaining
  laminectomy r.
Suarez r.
submucous r.
Sugita r.
suprapubic self-retaining r.
surgical r.
Sweeney posterior vaginal
  r.

retractor (*continued*)
    Sweet amputation r.
    sweetheart r.
    Symmonds hysterectomy r.
    sympathectomy r.
    T-bar r.
    T-model endaural r.
    table-fixed r.
    Tang r.
    TARA retropubic r.
    Taylor Britetrac r.
    Taylor fiberoptic r.
    Taylor spinal r.
    Tebbets ribbon r.
    Teflon iris r.
    Temple-Fay laminectomy r.
    Tepas r.
    Terino facial implant r.
    Tew cranial r.
    Tew spinal r.
    Theis self-retaining rib r.
    Theis vein r.
    Thoma tissue r.
    Thomas r.
    Thompson r.
    Thorlakson deep
      abdominal r.
    Thorlakson multipurpose r.
    Thornton iris r.
    three-prong rake blade r.
    thumb r.
    Thurmond iris r.
    thymus r.
    thyroid r.
    tibial r.
    Tiko pliable iris r.
    Tiko rake r.
    Tillary double-ended r.
    tissue r.
    titanium wound r.
    Toennis r.
    tongue r.
    tonsillar pillar r.
    toothed r.
    Tower interchangeable r.
    Tower rib r.
    Tower spinal r.
    tracheal r.

retractor (*continued*)
    transconjunctival r.
    transoral r.
    Trent eye r.
    trigeminal self-retaining r.
    Tubinger self-retaining r.
    Tucker-Levine vocal cord r.
    Tuffier abdominal r.
    Tuffier rib r.
    Tuffier-Raney laminectomy
      r.
    Tupper hand-holder and r.
    Turner-Doyen r.
    Turner-Warwick posterior
      urethral r.
    Turner-Warwick prostate r.
    two-prong rake r.
    Tyrer nerve root r.
    Tyrrell hook r.
    U-shaped r.
    U. S. Army double-ended r.
    Ullrich self-retaining
      laminectomy r.
    Ullrich-St. Gallen
      self-retaining r.
    umbrella r.
    Universal r.
    Upper Hands self-retaining
      r.
    upper-lateral exposing r.
    Urban r.
    USA r.
    uvular r.
    Vacher self-retaining r.
    vacuum r.
    vaginal r.
    vagotomy r.
    Vail lid r.
    Vaiser-Cibis muscle r.
    Valin hemilaminectomy
      self-retaining r.
    Vasco-Posada orbital r.
    vascular spring r.
    Veenema retropubic
      self-retaining r.
    vein hook r.
    ventriculogram r.
    Verbrugge r.

retractor (*continued*)

vertical self-retaining bone r.
vesical r.
vessel r.
Viboch iliac graft r.
Villalta r.
Vinke r.
Visitec iris r.
Volkmann finger r.
Volkmann hand r.
Volkmann pocket r.
Volkmann rake r.
W. D. Johnson epicardial r.
Wachtenfeldt-Stille r.
Walden-Aufricht nasal r.
Walker gallbladder r.
Walker lid r.
Walter nasal r.
Walter-Deaver r.
Wangensteen r.
Weary nerve root r.
Webb r.
Webb-Balfour self-retaining abdominal r.
Webster abdominal r.
Weder r.
Weder-Solenberger pillar r.
Weder-Solenberger tonsillar r.
weighted posterior r.
Weinberg "Joe's hoe" double-ended r.
Weinberg vagotomy r.
Weinstein horizontal r.
Weinstein intestinal r.
Weitlaner brain r.
Weitlaner hinged r.
Weitlaner microsurgery r.
Weitlaner self-retaining r.
Wellington Hospital vaginal r.
Welsh iris r.
Wesson perineal self-retaining r.
Wesson vaginal r.
Wexler abdominal r.

retractor (*continued*)

Wexler deep-spreader blade abdominal r.
Wexler large-frame abdominal r.
Wexler lateral side-blade abdominal r.
Wexler malleable-blade abdominal r.
Wexler self-retaining r.
Wexler Universal joint abdominal r.
Wexler vaginal r.
Wexler X-P large abdominal r.
Wexler-Balfour r.
Wexler-Bantam r.
White-Lillie r.
White-Proud uvular r.
Wichman r.
Wieder dental r.
Wieder pillar r.
Wieder-Solenberger pillar r.
Wiet r.
Wigderson ribbon r.
Wilder scleral self-retaining r.
Wilkes self-retaining r.
Wilkinson abdominal r.
Wilkinson ring-frame abdominal r.
Wilkinson self-retaining abdominal r.
Wilkinson-Deaver blade abdominal r.
Willauer-Deaver r.
Williams microlumbar r.
Williams rod self-retaining r.
Wills eye lacrimal r.
Wilmer cryosurgical iris r.
Wilmer iris r.
Wilmer-Bagley r.
Wilson r.
Wiltse iliac r.
Wiltse-Bankart r.
Wiltse-Gelpi self-retaining r.
Winsburg-White r.

retractor (*continued*)
   wiring r.
   Wise orbital r.
   Wolf meniscal r.
   Wolfson gallbladder r.
   Woodward r.
   Worrall deep r.
   Wort antral r.
   Wullstein self-retaining ear
      r.
   Wullstein-Weitlaner
      self-retaining r.
   Wylie renal vein r.
   Wylie splanchnic r.
   Yasargil r.
   Yasargil-Leyla brain r.
   Young anterior prostatic r.
   Young bifid r.
   Young bladder r.
   Young bulb r.
   Young lateral prostatic r.
   Young prostatic r.
   Yu-Holtgrewe prostatic r.
   Z r.
   Zalkind lung r.
   Zalkind-Balfour
      center-blade r.
   Zalkind-Balfour
      self-retaining r.
   Zenker r.
   Zimberg esophageal hiatal
      r.
   Zylik-Michaels r.

Reuter
   R. bobbin tube
   R. suprapubic cannula
   R. suprabubic trocar

Revelation
   R. endocardial
      microcatheter
   R. hip system
   R. Tx microcatheter

Revo
   R. retrievable cancellous
      screw
   R. rotator cuff repair system

Rhino Rocket nasal packing

Rhyder diagnostic catheter

Rigiflex TTS balloon catheter

Ring hip prosthesis

RITA ablation catheter

Rivas vascular catheter

Riza-Ribe grasper needle

Robicsek vascular probe

ROC
   R. suture fastener
   R. XS suture fastener

Rochester bone trephine

rod
   Acufex TAG r.
   Biofix absorbable r.

Roeder loop

Rogozinski spinal fixation
   system

RollerLOOP

Romano surgical curved drilling
   system

rongeur
   FlexTip intervertebral r.

Rosenkranz pediatric retractor
   system

Rosen needle

Rotablator
   R. RotaLink rotational
      atherectomy device
   R. RotaLink Plus rotational
      atheterectomy device

Roth Grip-Tip suture guide

Rothman Gilbard corneal punch

Roticulator stapler

Roy-Camille plate

Ruiz-Cohen round expander

Ruiz microkeratome

Rumi uterine manipulator

Russell-Taylor nail

Russian forceps

Rutkow
    R. sutureless plug
    R. sutureless patch

RX
    RX Herculink biliary stent
        system
    RX Multi-Link coronary
        stent system

Saber
    S. ArthroWand
    S. BT blunt-tip surgical
      trocar

Sable PTCA balloon catheter

Sabreloc
    S. spatula needle
    S. suture

Sadowsky hook wire

Safetex cervical spatula

Sahli needle

Sandoz
    S. balloon replacement
      tube
    S. Caluso PEG
    S. suction tube

SatinCrescent
    S. implant knife
    S. tunneler

SatinShortcut ophthalmic knife

SatinSlit keratome

Sauvage
    S. Bionit graft
    S. Dacron graft
    S. fabric graft prosthesis
    S. filamentous prosthesis
    S. filamentous velour graft

scalpel
    Harmonic s.
    Hemostatix s.
    Shaw s.
    Smart s.
    stone-age s.

Schneider
    S. catheter
    S. driver-extractor
    S. Magic Wallstent
    S. PTCA instruments
    S. rod
    S. self-broaching pin
    S. Wallstent

scissors
    Adson-Toennis s.
    Bellucci s.
    Castanares face-lift s.
    Electroscope s.
    Evershears II bipolar
      curved s.
    F. L. Fischer bayonet s.
    Harvester bipolar s.
    Lloyd-Davies s.
    Twisk s.
    Z-scissors

Scorpio total knee system

Scoville retractor

screw
    Absolute absorbable s.
    Acutrak s.
    alar s.
    s. alignment bar
    s. alignment rod
    Alta cancellous s.
    Alta cortical s.
    Alta cross-locking s.
    Alta lag s.
    Alta supracondylar s.
    Alta transverse s.
    amputation s.
    anchor s.
    Arthrex sheathed
      interference s.
    Asnis 2 guided s.
    Asnis guided s.
    Asnis III cannulated s.
    Aten olecranon s.
    Barouk cannulated bone s.
    Basile hip s.
    bicortical superior border s.
    bioabsorbable interference s.
    Biofix absorbable s.
    biointerference s.
    Biologically Quiet
      interference s.
    Biologically Quiet
      reconstruction s.

screw (*continued*)

Bionix self-reinforced PLLA
smart s.
BioSorb endoscopic
browlift s.
Bone Mulch s.
bone s.
Bosworth coracoclavicular
s.
brow lift suspension s.
Buttress thread s.
Calcitek retaining s.
Camino subdural s.
cancellous bone s.
cannulated cancellous lag
s.
Carol Gerard s.
carpal scaphoid s.
Carrel-Girard s.
Caspar cervical s.
Clearfix meniscal s.
Cohort bone s.
Collison s.
compression hip screw
CHS
s. compressor
Concise compression hip s.
cortex s.
cortical s.
Cotrel pedicle s.
cover s.
craniomaxillofacial s.
Crites laryngeal cotton s.
crown drill s.
cruciate head bone s.
cruciform head bone s.
Cubbins s.
Demuth hip s.
dental implant cover s.
Dentatus s.
s. depth calibrator
s. depth gauge
DePuy interference s.
Deyerle s.
distal locking s.
distraction s.
Doyen myoma s.
Doyen tumor s.

screw (*continued*)

Duo-Drive cortical s.
Dwyer spinal s.
dynamic condylar s.
dynamic hip s.
Edwards sacral s.
Eggers s.
encased s.
endocardial s.
EndoFix absorbable
interference s.
expansion s.
Fabian s.
Fixateur Interne s.
fixation s.
foreign body s.
four-tap s.
Geckeler s.
Gentle Threads interference
s.
Glasser fixation s.
glenoid fixation s.
s. grip
Guardsman femoral
interference s.
Hahn s.
Hall spinal s.
Hall-Morris biphase s.
healing s.
Heck s.
Herbert bone s.
Herbert scaphoid s.
Herbert-Whipple bone s.
Howmedica Universal
compression s.
iliac s.
iliosacral s.
Ilizarov s.
ImplaMed gold s.
Implant Innovations
titanium s.
Implant Support Systems
titanium s.
Instrument Makar
biodegradable
interference s.
Integrity acetabular cup s.
interference s.

screw (*continued*)
  interfragmentary lag s.
  intracranial pressure
    monitor s.
  Isola spinal implant system
    iliac s.
  Isola vertebral s.
  Jeter lag s.
  Jeter position s.
  Jewett pickup s.
  Johannson lag s.
  Johannson-Stille lag s.
  KLS Centre-Drive s.
  KLS-Martin Centre-Drive s.
  Kostuik s.
  Kristiansen eyelet lag s.
  Kurosaka interference-fit s.
  lag s.
  Lane bone s.
  lateral s.
  Leibinger Micro Plus s.
  Leibinger Mini Würzburg s.
  Leibinger Würzburg s.
  Leinbach olecranon s.
  Leone expansion s.
  Lewis tonsillar s.
  Lindorf lag s.
  Lindorf position s.
  Linvatec absorbable s.
  Linvatec bioabsorbable
    interference s.
  locking s.
  Lorenz s.
  Luhr implant s.
  Luhr Vitallium s.
  lumbar pedicle s.
  Lundholm s.
  Luque II s.
  mandibular angle fracture
    intraoral open reduction s.
  Marion s.
  maxillofacial bone s.
  McLaughlin carpal
    scaphoid s.
  medial bicortical s.
  medial unicortical s.
  metallic s.
  Micro Plus s.

screw (*continued*)
  Mille Pattes s.
  mini lag s.
  mini Würzburg s.
  monocortical s.
  Morris biphase s.
  multiaxial s.
  myoma s.
  navicular s.
  Neufeld s.
  No-Lok compression s.
  Nobelpharma gold
    prosthetic retaining s.
  s. occlusive clamp
  Olerud PSF s.
  Omega compression hip s.
  oral s.
  Orion plate and s.
  Orthex cannulated titanium
    bone s.
  Orthofix s.
  orthopedic s.
  Osteomed s.
  Palex expansion s.
  pedicle s.
  PerFixation s.
  Periotest Implant
    Innovations gold s.
  Phantom interference s.
  Phillips recessed-head s.
  Pilot point s.
  polyaxial cervical s.
  polylactide absorbable s.
  pretapped Synthes lag s.
  Pro/Pel cannulated
    interference s.
  pull s.
  Quiet interference s.
  Reddick-Saye s.
  resorbable plate and s.
  ReUnite orthopedic s.
  reverse-threaded s.
  Revo retrievable cancellous
    s.
  Richards classic
    compression hip s.
  Richmond subarachnoid s.
  rigid pedicle s.

screw (*continued*)
    Rockwood shoulder s.
    Russell-Taylor s.
    sacral alar s.
    sacral pedicle s.
    Salzburg s.
    Scuderi s.
    self-tapping bone s.
    self-tapping Leibinger lag s.
    set s.
    Sharpey s.
    Sherman bone s.
    silk s.
    Simmons double-hole
        spinal s.
    Simmons-Martin s.
    SmartScrew s.
    Smith & Nephew s.
    Spiessel lag s.
    Spiessel position s.
    stainless steel s.
    Steinhauser lag s.
    Steinhauser position s.
    step s.
    Stryker lag s.
    subarachnoid s.
    superior thoracic pedicle s.
    superlag s.
    syndesmotic s.
    Synthes compression hip s.
    Synthes s.
    s. tap
    Texas Scottish Rite Hospital
        pedicle s.
    Thatcher s.
    thoracolumbar pedicle s.
    ThreadLoc driver mount s.
    ThreadLoc retaining s.
    Ti alloy s.
    TiMesh s.
    titanium s.
    tonsillar s.
    Townley bone graft s.
    Townsend-Gilfillan s.
    TPS-coated s.
    traction tongs s.
    transarticular s.
    transfixion s.

screw (*continued*)
    transpedicular s.
    triangulated pedicle s.
    tulip pedicle s.
    tumor s.
    Venable s.
    Vilex cannulated s.
    Virgin hip s.
    Vitallium s.
    Weise jack s.
    Wood s.
    Woodruff s.
    Yuan s.
    Zielke s.
    Zimmer s.

Secu clip

Secur-Fit hip system

Seidel
    S. humeral locking nail
    S. intramedullary fixation

Seitzinger tripolar cutting
    forceps

Selector ultrasonic aspirator

Selute
    S. Picotip steroid-eluting
        lead
    S. steroid-eluting lead

Selverstone clamp

Senning intra-atrial baffle

Sepracoat coating solution

Seprafilm bioresorbable
    embrane

Sepramesh biosurgical
    composite

SET three-lumen thrombectomy
    catheter

Sewell retractor

Shah permanent ventilating
    tube

Shaldon catheter

Shaw scalpel

Shikani middle meatal
   antrostomy stent

Shirley wound drain

ShortCut knife

shunt
   Allen-Brown vascular
      access s.
   Anastaflo intervascular s.
   Buselmeier s.
   Cordis-Hakim s.
   Denver pleuroperitoneal s.
   Flo-Thru s.
   Gibson inner ear s.
   Gott s.
   Holter s.
   House and pulec otic-
      periotic s
   Kasai peritoneal venous s.
   LeVeen peritoneal s.
   Orbis-Sigma s.
   Pruitt-Inahara carotid s.
   Quinton-Scribner s.
   Ramirez s.
   Rivetti-Levinson
      intraluminal s.
   T-AnastaFlo s.
   Thomas vascular access s.
   TIPSS s.
   Torkildsen s.
   Vitagraft arteriovenous s.
   Warren splenorenal s.
   Winters s.

Shur-Strip sterile wound closure
   tape

Shutt-Mantis retrograde forceps

SignaDress hydrocolloid
   dressing material

Silon tent

Silverlon wound packing
   strips

Simpson
   S. atherectomy catheter

Simpson (*continued*)
   S. Coronary AtheroCath
      system
   S. peripheral AtheroCath

SinuSeal resorbable nasal
   packing

Sine-U-View nasal endoscope

Sinskey hook

SiteGuard MVP transparent
   adhesive film dressing

Skimmer RRP laryngeal shaver

Skinny
   S. dilatation catheter
   S. needle

Skin Skribe skin marker

SkinTegrity hydrogel dressing

sling
   Straight-In male s.
   Stratasis urethral s.
   SurgiSis s.
   Suspend s.
   triangular vaginal patch s.
   UltraSling s.

Slinky catheter

SmallPort needle

SmartNeedle

Smithwick hook

snare
   BiSNARE bipolar
      polypectomy s.

Soehendra
   S. dilator
   S. stent retriever

Soft N Dry Merocel sponge

Soft Shield collagen corneal
   shield

Soft Torque uterine catheter

Sof-Wick

Sof-Wick (*continued*)
  S. drain sponges
  S. dressing

Solcotrans
  S. closed vacuum-drainage
    system
  S. drainage/reinfusion
    system

Solera thrombectomy catheter

Solitaire needle

Solo catheter with Pro/Pel
  coating

SoloPass stent/catheter

SoloSite
  S. nonsterile hydrogel
    wound dressing
  S. wound gel

Somer uterine elevator

Somjee-Crabtree temporal bone
  support clamp

Somnus probe

Sonde enteroscope

Sones catheter

Sonolith Praktis lithotripter

Sorbsan topical wound dressing

Spacekeeper retractor

Spacemaker balloon dissector

Space-OR flexible internal
  retractor

speculum
  adolescent vaginal s.
  Adson s.
  Agrikola eye s.
  Alfonso eyelid s.
  Allen-Heffernan nasal s.
  Allingham rectal s.
  Amko vaginal s.
  anal s.
  s. anoscope

speculum (*continued*)
  Arruga eye s.
  Arruga globe s.
  Artisan wide-angle vaginal
    s.
  Aufricht septal s.
  aural s.
  Auvard Britetrac s.
  Auvard weighted vaginal s.
  Auvard-Remine vaginal s.
  Azar lid s.
  Bárány s.
  Barr anal s.
  Barr rectal s.
  Barr-Shuford s.
  Barraquer eye s.
  Barraquer solid s.
  Barraquer wire s.
  Barraquer-Colibri eye s.
  Barraquer-Douvas eye s.
  Barraquer-Floyd s.
  basket-style scleral
    supporter s.
  Beard eye s.
  Becker-Park s.
  Beckman nasal s.
  Beckman-Colver nasal s.
  Bedrossian eye s.
  Bercovici wire lid s.
  Berens eye s.
  Berlind-Auvard vaginal s.
  Bionix nasal s.
  bivalved anal s.
  blackened s.
  Bodenheimer rectal s.
  Bosworth nasal wire s.
  Boucheron ear s.
  Bovin vaginal s.
  Bovin-Stille vaginal s.
  Bowman eye s.
  Bozeman s.
  Braun s.
  Breisky vaginal s.
  Breisky-Navratil vaginal s.
  Breisky-Stille s.
  Brewer vaginal s.
  Brinkerhoff rectal s.
  Britetrac s.

speculum (*continued*)
  Bronson s.
  Bronson-Park s.
  Bronson-Turtz s.
  Brown ear s.
  Bruening s.
  Bruner vaginal s.
  Buie-Smith rectal s.
  Burnett Sani-Spec
    disposable s.
  Callahan modification s.
  Carpel s.
  Carter septal s.
  Caspar s.
  Castallo eye s.
  Castroviejo eye s.
  Chelsea-Eaton anal s.
  Chevalier Jackson laryngeal
    s.
  Clark eye s.
  Coakley nasal s.
  Collin vaginal s.
  Converse nasal s.
  Conway lid s.
  Cook eye s.
  Cook rectal s.
  Cottle nasal s.
  Cottle septal s.
  Critchett eye s.
  Culler iris s.
  Cusco vaginal s.
  Cushing-Landolt
    transsphenoidal s.
  Czerny rectal s.
  David rectal s.
  DeLee s.
  DeRoaldes s.
  Desmarres eye s.
  Desmarres lid s.
  DeVilbiss vaginal s.
  DeVilbiss-Stacy s.
  Disposo-Spec disposable s.
  Docherty cheek s.
  Douglas mucosal s.
  Douvas-Barraquer s.
  Downes nasal s.
  Doyen vaginal s.
  duckbill s.

speculum (*continued*)
  Dudley-Smith rectal s.
  Duplay nasal s.
  Duplay-Lynch nasal s.
  Dynacor vaginal s.
  ear s.
  Eaton nasal s.
  Eisenhammer s.
  endaural s.
  ENT s.
  Erhardt ear s.
  Erosa-Spec vaginal s.
  eye s.
  Fansler rectal s.
  Fanta s.
  Farkas urethral s.
  Farrior ear s.
  Farrior oval s.
  Fergusson tubular vaginal s.
  fiberoptic vaginal s.
  fine-wire s.
  Flannery ear s.
  flat-bladed nasal s.
  Flint glass s.
  Floyd-Barraquer wire s.
  Forbes esophageal s.
  s. forceps
  Foster-Ballenger nasal s.
  four-prong finger s.
  Fox eye s.
  Fränkel s.
  Gaffee s.
  Garrigue weighted vaginal
    s.
  Gerzog nasal s.
  Gilbert-Graves s.
  Gleason s.
  Goldbacher anoscope s.
  Goldstein septal s.
  Goligher s.
  Graefe eye s.
  Graves bivalve s.
  Graves Britetrac vaginal s.
  Graves Coldlite s.
  Graves open-side vaginal s.
  Gruber ear s.
  Guild-Pratt rectal s.
  Guilford-Wright bivalve s.

speculum (*continued*)
  Guist s.
  Guist-Black eye s.
  Guist-Bloch s.
  Gutter s.
  Guttmann vaginal s.
  Guyton-Maumenee s.
  Guyton-Park eye s.
  Gyn-A-Lite vaginal s.
  Haglund vaginal s.
  Haglund-Stille vaginal s.
  Halle infant nasal s.
  Halle-Tieck nasal s.
  Hardy bivalve s.
  Hardy nasal bivalve s.
  Hardy-Duddy s.
  Hartmann dewaxer s.
  Hartmann ear s.
  Hartmann nasal s.
  Hayes vaginal s.
  Heffernan nasal s.
  Helmholtz s.
  Helmont s.
  Henrotin weighted vaginal s.
  Hertel nephrostomy s.
  Higbee vaginal s.
  Hinkle-James rectal s.
  Hirschman anoscope rectal s.
  s. holder
  Holinger infant esophageal s.
  Hood-Graves vaginal s.
  Hough-Boucheron ear s.
  House stapes s.
  Huffman infant vaginal s.
  Huffman-Graves adolescent vaginal s.
  Huffman-Graves vaginal s.
  Iliff-Park s.
  illuminated s.
  s. illuminator
  Ingals nasal s.
  Ives rectal s.
  Jackson vaginal s.
  Jaffe eyelid s.
  Jarit-Graves vaginal s.

speculum (*continued*)
  Jarit-Pederson vaginal s.
  Jonas-Graves vaginal s.
  Kahn-Graves vaginal s.
  Kaiser s.
  Kalinowski ear s.
  Kalinowski-Verner ear s.
  Katena s.
  Keeler-Pierse eye s.
  Keizer-Lancaster eye s.
  Kelly rectal s.
  Killian nasal s.
  Killian rectal s.
  Killian septal s.
  Killian-Halle nasal s.
  Klaff septal s.
  KleenSpec disposable vaginal s.
  Knapp eye s.
  Knapp-Culler s.
  Knolle lens s.
  Kogan endocervical s.
  Kogan urethra s.
  Kramer ear s.
  Kratz aspirating s.
  Kratz-Barraquer wire lid s.
  Kristeller vaginal s.
  Kyle nasal s.
  Lancaster eye s.
  Lancaster lid s.
  Lancaster-O'Connor s.
  Landau s.
  Lang eye s.
  Lawford s.
  LeFort s.
  Lempert-Beckman-Colver endaural s.
  Lempert-Colver endaural s.
  Lester-Burch eye s.
  lid s.
  LidFix s.
  Lieberman aspirating s.
  Lieberman K-Wire s.
  lighted s.
  Lillie nasal s.
  Lindstrom-Chu aspirating s.
  Lister-Burch cyc s.
  Lofberg vaginal s.

speculum (*continued*)
  Lucae ear s.
  Luer eye s.
  McBratney aspirating s.
  Machat adjustable
    aspirating wire s.
  McHugh oval s.
  McKee s.
  McKinney eye s.
  McLaughlin s.
  Macon Hospital s.
  McPherson eye s.
  Mahoney intranasal antral s.
  Manche LASIK s.
  Martin rectal s.
  Martin vaginal s.
  Mason-Auvard weighted
    vaginal s.
  Mathews rectal s.
  Matzenauer vaginal s.
  Maumenee-Park eye s.
  Mayer s.
  Mellinger eye s.
  Mellinger fenestrated
    blades s.
  Mellinger-Axenfeld eye s.
  Merz-Vienna nasal s.
  Metcher eye s.
  Miller vaginal s.
  Milligan s.
  Montgomery vaginal s.
  Montgomery-Bernstine s.
  Moria one-piece s.
  Mosher nasal s.
  Mosher urethral s.
  Moynihan s.
  Mueller eye s.
  Muir rectal s.
  Murdock eye s.
  Murdock-Wiener eye s.
  Murdoon eye s.
  Myles nasal s.
  Myles-Ray s.
  Nasa-Spec nasal s.
  nasal bivalve s.
  nasopharyngeal s.
  National ear s.
  National Graves vaginal s.

speculum (*continued*)
  Nott vaginal s.
  Nott-Gutmann vaginal s.
  Noyes s.
  Omni-Park s.
  one-hand s.
  open-side vaginal s.
  O'Sullivan-O'Connor vaginal
    s.
  oval s.
  Pannu-Kratz-Barraquer s.
  Park eye s.
  Park-Guyton eye s.
  Park-Guyton-Callahan eye
    s.
  Park-Guyton-Maumenee s.
  Park-Maumenee s.
  Parks anal s.
  Patton septal s.
  Pearce eye s.
  Pederson vaginal s.
  pediatric lid s.
  pediatric s.
  Pennington rectal s.
  Picot vaginal s.
  Pierse eye s.
  Pilling-Hartmann s.
  plain wire s.
  Politzer ear s.
  post-urethroplasty review s.
  Pratt bivalve s.
  Pratt rectal s.
  Preefer eye s.
  Prima Series LEEP s.
  Prospec disposable s.
  Proud infant turbinate s.
  Pynchon nasal s.
  Rappazzo s.
  Ray nasal s.
  rectal s.
  Reipen s.
  Relat vaginal s.
  reversible lid s.
  Rica ear s.
  Rica nasal septal s.
  Rica vaginal s.
  Richard Gruber s.
  Richnau-Holmgren ear s.

speculum (*continued*)
>Roberts esophageal s.
>Roberts oval s.
>Rosenthal urethral s.
>round s.
>Sani-Spec vaginal s.
>Sato s.
>Sauer eye s.
>Sauer infant eye s.
>Saunders eye s.
>Sawyer rectal s.
>Schweizer s.
>Scott ear s.
>Semb vaginal s.
>Senturia pharyngeal s.
>Serdarevic s.
>Seyfert vaginal s.
>Shea s.
>shoehorn s.
>Siegle ear s.
>Simcoe eye s.
>Simcoe wire s.
>Simcoe-Barraquer eye s.
>Simmonds vaginal s.
>Simrock s.
>Sims double-ended vaginal s.
>Sims rectal s.
>Sims vaginal s.
>Sisson-Cottle s.
>Sisson-Vienna s.
>Sluder sphenoidal s.
>SMIC ear s.
>SMIC nasal septal s.
>Smirmaul eyelid s.
>Smith anal s.
>Smith eye s.
>Smith-Buie rectal s.
>Sonnenschein nasal s.
>stapes s.
>Stearnes s.
>Steiner-Auvard s.
>Stop eye s.
>Storz nasal s.
>Storz septal s.
>Storz-Vienna nasal s.
>Sutherland-Grieshaber s.
>Sweeney posterior vaginal s.

speculum (*continued*)
>Swiss-pattern s.
>Swolin self-retaining vaginal s.
>Tauber s.
>Taylor vaginal s.
>Terson s.
>Thornton open-wire lid s.
>Thudichum nasal s.
>Tieck nasal s.
>Tieck-Halle infant nasal s.
>Torchia eye s.
>Toynbee ear s.
>s. transilluminator
>transsphenoidal s.
>Trelat vaginal s.
>Troeltsch ear s.
>Turner-Warwick post-urethroplasty review s.
>Ullrich vaginal s.
>Universal s.
>vaginal s.
>Vaginard metal s.
>Vauban s.
>Verner s.
>Verner-Kalinowski s.
>Vernon-David rectal s.
>Vienna Britetrac nasal s.
>Voltolini nasal s.
>Vu-Max vaginal s.
>Watson s.
>Weeks eye s.
>weighted vaginal s.
>Weiner s.
>Weisman-Graves open-sided vaginal s.
>Weiss s.
>Weissbarth vaginal s.
>Welch Allyn illuminated s.
>Welch Allyn KleenSpec vaginal s.
>Wellington Hospital vaginal s.
>Wiener eye s.
>Williams eye s.
>Wilson-Kirbe s.
>wire bivalve vaginal s.
>wire lid s.

speculum (*continued*)
  Worcester City Hospital s.
  Yankauer nasopharyngeal s.
  Ziegler eye s.
  Zower s.
  Zylik-Michaels s.

Speedy balloon catheter

Sperma-Tex preshaped mesh

Spiessel
  S. internal screw fixation
  S. lag screw
  S. position screw

SpiraStent ureteral stent

SpiroFlo bioabsorbable prostate stent

splint
  AirFlex carpal tunnel
  Brooke Army Hospital s.
  Breathe-Easy nasal s.
  Budin toe s.
  Delbet s.
  Dennis Brown clubfoot s.
  Denver nasal s.
  Doyle Combo nasal airway s.
  Doyle Shark nasal s.
  Flexisplint
  Joint-Jack finger s.
  MindSet toe s.
  Radstat wrist s.
  Rolyan Gel Shell s.
  Slattery-McGrouther dynamic flexion s.
  Thomas s.
  Versi-Splint

sponge
  Actifoam collagen s.
  Actifoam hemostat s.
  Helistat absorbable collagen s.
  hemostatic s.
  K-sponge
  Lapwall laparotomy s.
  Merocel s.

sponge (*continued*)
  peanut s.
  Protectaid s.
  Ray-Tec x-ray detectable surgical s.
  Sof-Wick s.
  Taka microneurosurgical s.
  Vistec x-ray detectable s.
  Weck-cel s.

sponge dissector

spoon forceps

SprayGel adhesion barrier system

Sprint catheter with Pro/Pel coating

Spyglass angiography catheter

STAAR
  S. implantable contact lens
  S. Toric implantable contact lens

Stability total hip system

Stableloc II external fixator system

Stadler's splint

Stamey needle

Stamey-Malecot catheter

Stammberger antrum punch

stapler
  Auto Suture Multifire Endo GIA 30 s.
  Auto Suture Premium CEEA s.
  Cobe gun s.
  EEA s.
  Endo-GIA suture s.
  Endo-Hernia s.
  Endopath EMS hernia s.
  ILA s.
  Multifire Endo GIA s.
  Multifire GIA s.
  Multifire VersaTack s.

stapler (*continued*)
    PolyGIA s.
    Premium CEEA circular s.
    Proximate flexible linear s.
    Proximate linear cutter s.
    Roticulator s.
    SDsorb E-Z tac system
    SDsorb meniscal s.
    SQS-20 subcuticular skin s.
    Surgeon's Choice s.
    TL-90 s.

Starion thermal cautery hook

STARR
    S. Glaucoma Wick
    S. implantable contact lens
    S. low-diopter intraocular
      lens
    S. Toric intraocular lens

Statak soft tissue attachment
    device

StaLock Universal Plus suture-
    free anchor

Steffee
    S. plate
    S. screw

Steinhauser
    S. internal screw fixation
    S. lag screw
    S. position screw

Stelid II pacing lead

Stelix pacing lead

Steinmann pin

stem

Steis needle
    AcuMatch L series
      cemented femoral s.

stent
    Acculink self-expanding s.
    ACS OTW HP coronary
    ACS Rx Multi-Link coronary
      s.
    ACT-one coronary s.

stent (*continued*)
    activated balloon
      expandable intravascular s.
    AneuRx aortic aneurysm
      stent-graft
    AngioStent cardiovascular
      s.
    Atkinson tube s.
    balloon expandable s.
    Bard Memotherm
      colorectal s.
    Bard XT coronary s.
    BeStent
    BeStent2 laser-cut s.
    BiodivYsio s.
    BioSorb resorbable urology
      s.
    Bx Velocity sirolimus-
      coated s.
    CardioCoil coronary s.
    CarotidCoil s.
    Champion s.
    Cragg Endopro System I s.
    CrossFlex LC coronary s.
    Crown s.
    DISA S-flex coronary s.
    Dua s
    Dumon tracheobronchial s.
    Dynalink 0.035 biliary self-
      expanding s.
    Elastalloy Ultraflex Strecker
      nitinol s.
    ENDOcare nitinol s.
    Endocare Horizon prostatic
      s.
    EndoCoil biliary s.
    Enforcer SDS coronary s.
    EsophaCoil self-expanding
      esophageal s.
    Express s.
    Fader Tip ureteral s.
    Focustent coronary s.
    gfx s.
    Gianturco expandable
      metallic biliary s.
    Gianturco-Rosch Z-stent
    Gianturco-Roubin flexible
      coil s.

stent (*continued*)
Gianturco-Roubin s.
Guidant Multi-Link Tetra
coronary s.
Harrell Y s.
Hepamed-coated
Wiktor s.
Hood stoma s.
Horizon s.
InStent Carotid Coil s.
IntraCoil nitinol s.
IntraStent DoubleStrut
biliary endoprosthesis
INX stainless steel s.
IRIS coronary s.
Jostent s.
Lubri-Flex s.
Luminexx biliary s.
Magic Wallstent
Medtronic S7 coronary s.
Megalink biliary s.
Memotherm colorectal s.
Memotherm endoscopic
biliary s.
Memotherm nitanol s.
MeroGel sinus s.
Mini Crown s.
Multi-Flex s.
Multi-Link Pixel s.
Multilink Duet s.
NexStent carotid s.
NIR Elite over-the-wire s.
NIR ON Ranger
premounted s.
NIR paclitaxel-coated
coronary s.
NIR Primo Monorail s.
NIR with SOX coronary s.
Niroyal Elite Monorail
coronary s.
Niroyal Monorail s.
nitinol mesh s.
OMNILINK biliary s.
OmniStent
paclitaxel-coated coronary
s.
Palmaz Corinthian
transhepatic biliary s.

stent (*continued*)
Palmaz-Schatz balloon-
expandable s.
Palmaz-Schatz Crown
balloon-expandable s.
Palmaz-Schatz Mini Crown
s.
Paragon Champion s.
Perflex stainless steel s.
Percuflex Plus s.
ProstaCoil self-expanding s.
Radius s.
RX Herculink Plus biliary s.
SAXX renal s.
Schneider Wallstent
Shikani middle meatal
antrostomy s.
S.M.A.R.T. s.
SoloPass s.
SpiraStent ureteral s.
SpiraFlo prostate s.
Strecker s.
Stryker s.
Supra G coronary s.
Symphony s.
Talent LPS endoluminal
stent-graft
Ultraflex s.
UroCoil s.
UroLume urethral s.
VascuCoil peripheral
vascular s.
Vistaflex s.
Wallstent
Westaby s.
Wiktor balloon expandable
coronary s.
Wiktor GX s.
XT radiopaque coronary s.
Z s.

stereotactic vacuum-assisted
biopsy device (SVAB)

Stifcore aspiration needle

stockings
CircAid elastic s.
Jobst s.

stockings (*continued*)
Sigvaris cmopression s.
T.E.D. s.
thigh-high embolic s.

Storz
S. cholangiograsper
S. infant bronchoscope
S. radial incision marker

StraightShot arterial cannula

Stratasorb composite wound dressing

Strecker stent

StrykeFlow
S. electrocautery probe
S. suction irrigator

Stryker
S. drain
S. illuminated retractor
S. microdebrider
S. MixEvac
S. stent
S. wedge suture anchor

Stylus cardiovascular suture

Suction Buster catheter

Summit Krumeich-Barraquer microkeratome

Sundt-Kees clip

Superblade

Superglue tissue adhesive

Super Pinky

Superstat hemostatic wound pad

Supramid suture

SureBite biopsy forceps

Sure-Closure

SurePress
S. absorbent padding
S. high-compression bandage

SureSite transparent adhesive film dressing

Suretac bioabsorbable shoulder fixation device

Surfit adhesive

Surgeon's Choice surgical stapling system

Surgical
S. No Bounce mallet
S. Nu-Knit
S. Simplex-P bone cement

Surgicel
S. hemostatic material
S. Nu-Knit

Surgidac braided polyester suture

Surgifoam absorbable gelatin sponge

SurgiLav Plus hydro debridement system

Surgilene monofilament polypropylene suture material

Surgilon braided nyulon suture material

Surg-I-Loop silicone loop

Surgiport disposable trocar

Surgipro prolene mesh

SurgiSis
S. mesh
S. sling

Surgi-Stim postsurgical therapy system

suture
Acier stainless steel s.
Acufex bioabsorbable Suretac s.
Acutrol s.
Alcon s.
already-threaded s.
aluminum-bronze wire s.

suture (*continued*)
American silk s.
Ancap braided silk s.
s. anchor
angiocatheter with looped
 polypropylene s.
arterial silk s.
S. Assistant
S. Assistant instrument
atraumatic braided silk s.
atraumatic chromic s.
Aureomycin s.
Auto Suture AS
Barraquer silk s.
bastard s.
basting s.
BioSorb s.
Biosyn s.
black braided nylon s.
black braided silk s.
black braided s.
black twisted s.
Blalock s.
blanket s.
blue twisted cotton s.
blue-black monofilament s.
bolster s.
Bondek absorbable s.
bone wax s.
Bozeman s.
braided Ethibond s.
braided Mersilene s.
braided Nurolon s.
braided nylon s.
braided polyamide s.
braided polyester s.
braided silk s.
braided Vicryl s.
braided wire s.
Bralon s.
bridle s.
bronze wire s.
Brown & Sharpe s. gauge
 (B&S s. gauge)
Bunnell wire pull-out s.
s. button
cable wire s.
capitonnage s.

suture (*continued*)
Caprolactam s.
cardinal s.
Cardioflon s.
Cardionyl s.
cardiovascular Prolene s.
cardiovascular silk s.
Carrel s.
s. carrier
catgut s.
celluloid linen s.
cervical s.
Chinese fingertrap s.
Chinese twisted silk s.
chloramine catgut s.
chromated catgut s.
chromic blue dyed s.
chromic catgut s.
chromic collagen s.
chromic gut s.
chromicized catgut s.
circular s.
circumcisional s.
s. clip forceps
coated polyester s.
coated Vicryl Rapide s.
cocoon thread s.
collagen absorbable s.
compound s.
Connell s.
coronal s.
cotton Deknatel s.
cotton nonabsorbable s.
Cottony Dacron hollow s.
cranial s.
CT1 s.
Cushing s.
s. cushion
Custodis s.
s. cutter
Czerny s.
Czerny-Lembert s.
Dacron bolstered s.
Dacron traction s.
Dafilon s.
Dagrofil s.
Davis-Geck s.
Degnon s.

suture (*continued*)
    Deklene polypropylene s.
    Deknatel silk s.
    delayed s.
    dermal s.
    Dermalene polyethylene s.
    Dermalon cuticular s.
    Dexon absorbable synthetic
      polyglycolic acid s.
    Dexon II s.
    Dexon Plus s.
    DG Softgut s.
    Docktor s.
    double right-angle s.
    double-armed s.
    double-running penetrating
      keratoplasty s.
    Dulox s.
    Dupuytren s.
    Edinburgh s.
    EEA Auto S.
    elastic s.
    Endo Knot s.
    Endoloop s.
    EPTFE vascular s.
    Equisetene s.
    Ethi-pack s.
    Ethibond polybutilate-
      coated polyester s.
    Ethibond polyester s.
    Ethicon micropoint s.
    Ethicon Sabreloc s.
    Ethicon silk s.
    Ethicon-Atraloc s.
    Ethiflex retention s.
    Ethilon nylon s.
    everting mattress s.
    expanded
      polytetrafluoroethylene
      (EPTFE) s.
    extrachromic s.
    figure-of-eight s.
    filament s.
    fine chromic s.
    fine silk s.
    fingertrap s.
    Flaxedil s.
    Flexitone s.

suture (*continued*)
    Flexon steel s.
    formaldehyde catgut s.
    Foster s.
    Fothergill s.
    Frater s.
    Frost s.
    Gély s.
    Gaillard-Arlt s.
    Gambee s.
    gastrointestinal surgical gut
      s.
    gastrointestinal surgical
      linen s.
    gastrointestinal surgical silk
      s.
    general closure s.
    GI pop-off silk s.
    Gillies horizontal dermal s.
    glue-in s.
    Gore-Tex s.
    gossamer silk s.
    Gould s.
    green braided s.
    green Mersilene s.
    green monofilament
      polyglyconate s.
    groove s.
    s. guide
    Gussenbauer s.
    gut s.
    guy s.
    guy-steading s.
    Guyton-Friedenwald s.
    Halsted mattress s.
    Heaney s.
    heavy monofilament s.
    heavy retention s.
    heavy silk retention s.
    heavy wire s.
    heavy-gauge s.
    helical s.
    hemostatic s.
    Herculon s.
    s. holder
    s. hole drill
    Horsley s.
    Hu-Friedy PermaSharp s.

suture (*continued*)
IKI catgut s.
India rubber s.
interrupted pledgeted s.
intraluminal s.
Investa s.
iodine catgut s.
iodized surgical gut s.
iodochromic catgut s.
Ivalon s.
Jobert de Lamballe s.
Küstner s.
Kal-Dermic s.
kangaroo tendon s.
Kessler-Kleinert s.
Kirschner s.
Krackow s.
lacidem s.
lambdoidal s.
lancet s.
s. lancet
Lang s.
Lapra-Ty s.
large-caliber nonabsorbable
    s.
lateral trap s.
lead s.
lead-shot tie s.
LeFort s.
Lembert s.
Ligapak s.
Linatrix s.
Lindner corneoscleral s.
linen s.
Linvatec meniscal
    BioStinger anchor s.
S. Lok device
Look s.
Lukens catgut s.
malar periosteum-SMAS
    flap fixation s.
Mannis s.
Marlex s.
Marshall V-s.
mattress s.
Maxam s.
Maxon absorbable s.
Mayo linen s.

suture (*continued*)
McCannel s.
McLean s.
Measuroll s.
Medrafil wire s.
Meigs s.
Mersilene braided
    nonabsorbable s.
Mersilk s.
mesh s.
metal band s.
metallic s.
Micrins microsurgical s.
Micro-Glide corneal s.
MicroMite anchor s.
micropoint s.
middle palatine s.
Millipore s.
Miralene s.
Monocryl poliglecaprone s.
monofilament absorbable s.
monofilament clear s.
monofilament green s.
monofilament nylon s.
monofilament
    polypropylene s.
monofilament skin s.
monofilament steel s.
monofilament wire s.
Monosof s.
multifilament steel s.
multistrand s.
nasofrontal s.
natural s.
Needle-Less S.
neurosurgical s.
Nissen s.
nonabsorbable surgical s.
Nurolon s.
nylon 66 s.
nylon monofilament s.
nylon retention s.
oiled silk s.
opaque wire s.
Ophthalon s.
Oyloidin s.
Pagenstecher linen thread
    s.

suture (*continued*)
- Palfyn s.
- Panacryl s.
- Panalok absorbable s.
- Pancoast s.
- Paré s.
- Parker-Kerr basting s.
- s. passer
- PDS II Endoloop s.
- PDS Vicryl s.
- Pearsall Chinese twisted s.
- Pearsall silk s.
- Perlon s.
- Perma-Hand braided silk s.
- PermaSharp PGA s.
- s. pickup hook
- s. pickup spatula
- pin s.
- pink twisted cotton s.
- plain catgut s.
- plain collagen s.
- plain gut s.
- plastic s.
- pledget s.
- pledgeted Ethibond s.
- pledgeted mattress s.
- poliglecaprone 25 s.
- polyamide s.
- polybutester s.
- Polydek s.
- polydioxanone suture PDS
- polyester fiber s.
- polyethylene s.
- polyfilament s.
- polygalactic acid s.
- polyglactin 910 s.
- polyglecaprone 25 s.
- polyglycolate s.
- polyglycolic acid s.
- polyglyconate s.
- polypropylene button s.
- Polysorb s.
- pop-off s.
- preplaced s.
- presphenoethmoid s.
- Prolene polypropylene s.
- Pronova s.
- Proxi-Strip s.

suture (*continued*)
- Pulvertaft s.
- Purlon s.
- PVB s.
- pyoktanin catgut s.
- pyroglycolic acid s.
- Quickert s.
- Ramsey County pyoktanin catgut s.
- Rankin s.
- Rapide wound s.
- RB1 s.
- reabsorbable s.
- Reo Macrodex s.
- ribbon gut s.
- s. ring
- rip-cord s.
- rubber s.
- running nylon penetrating keratoplasty s.
- Sabreloc s.
- Saenger s.
- safety-bolt s.
- Safil synthetic absorbable surgical s.
- serrated s.
- seton s.
- SH popoff s.
- Sharpoint ophthalmic microsurgical s.
- Shirodkar s.
- Shoch s.
- shotted s.
- Siemens PTCA open-heart s.
- silicone-treated surgical silk s.
- silk braided s.
- silk Mersilene s.
- silk nonabsorbable s.
- silk pop-off s.
- silk stay s.
- silk traction s.
- silkworm gut s.
- Silky Polydek s.
- silver s.
- silverized catgut s.
- Sims s.

suture (*continued*)
 single-armed s.
 single-running s.
 Snellen s.
 Sofsilk coated and braided s.
 Sofsilk nonabsorbable silk s.
 Softgut surgical chromic catgut s.
 s. spacer
 Spanish blue virgin silk s.
 SS s.
 stainless steel wire s.
 Stallard-Liegard s.
 steel mesh s.
 Sterna-Band self-locking s.
 sternal wire s.
 Sturmdorf s.
 Stylus cardiovascular s.
 subannular mattress s.
 subcutaneous s.
 subcuticular s.
 Supolene s.
 Supramid bridle collagen s.
 Supramid Extra s.
 Supramid lens implant s.
 Surgaloy metallic s.
 surgical chromic s.
 surgical gut s.
 surgical linen s.
 surgical silk s.
 surgical steel s.
 Surgicraft s.
 Surgidac s.
 Surgidev s.
 Surgigut s.
 Surgilar s.
 Surgilene blue monofilament polypropylene s.
 Surgiloid s.
 Surgilon braided nylon s.
 Surgilon monofilament polypropylene s.
 Surgilope s.
 SurgiMed s.
 Surgipro s.

suture (*continued*)
 Surgiset s.
 Sutupak s.
 Suturamid s.
 Sutureloop colposuspension s.
 S. Strip
 S. Strip Plus
 swaged s.
 swaged-on s.
 Swedgeon s.
 Swiss blue virgin silk s.
 synthetic absorbable s.
 Synthofil s.
 s. tag forceps
 tantalum wire monofilament s.
 Tapercut s.
 Teflon-coated Dacron s.
 Teflon-pledgeted s.
 tension-requiring s.
 tantalum wire tension s.
 Tevdek pledgeted s.
 Thermo-Flex s.
 Thiersch s.
 thread s.
 through-and-through reabsorbable s.
 through-the-wall mattress s.
 Ti-Cron s.
 tiger gut s.
 Tinel s.
 transfixion s.
 transosseous s.
 transscleral s.
 twisted cotton s.
 twisted dermal s.
 twisted linen s.
 twisted silk s.
 twisted virgin silk s.
 Tycron s.
 tympanomastoid s.
 Tyrrell-Gray s.
 UltraFix MicroMite anchor s.
 umbilical tape s.
 unabsorbable s.
 undyed s.
 vascular silk s.

suture (*continued*)
Verhoeff s.
S. VesiBand organizer
Vicryl pop-off s.
Vicryl Rapide s.
Vicryl SH s.
Vienna wire s.
virgin silk s.
Viro-Tec s.
white braided silk s.
white nylon s.
white twisted s.
wing s.
s. wire
s. wire–cutting scissors
wire Zytor s.

Sutureloop suture

Suture Strip Plus

Swartz SL Series Fast-Cath
introducer

Swenson papillotome

Symphony stent

Synchro neurovascular guide
wire

Syntel latex-free embolectomy
catheter

Synthes
S. CerviFix system
S. compression hip screw
S. dorsal distal radius plate
S. drill
S. mini-L-plate
S. transbuccal trocar
S. Schuhli implant system
S. universal spine system

syringe
Accuguide s.
Bruening s.

system
Abbott. LifeCare PCA Plus II
infusion system
Abbott Lifeshield
needleless system

system (*continued*)
Abbott Plum infusion
system
ABG cement-free hip
system
Above-Knee Suction
Enhancement system
Acryl-X orthopaedic cement
removal system
Acucair continuous airflow
system
advanced breast biopsy
instrumentation system
(ABBI)
Accunet embolic protection
system
Accurus vitrectomy system
AccuTrack eye-tracking
system
Ancure system
AngioJet rheolytic
thrombectomy system
Apollo hip system
Apollo knee system
Beta-Cath system
Checkmate intravascular
brachytherapy system
COGNIShunt CNS fluid
shunt system
Cryocare cardiac surgical
system
Endocinch suturing system
Envoy middle ear
implantable system
HydroThermAblator system
Intrabeam system
Microvascular Anastomotic
Coupler System
Navitrack computer-
assisted system
Oasis sheet introducer
system
Oasis thrombectomy
system
OrthoPAT autotransfusion
system
Reflex anterior cervical
plate (ACP) system

system (*continued*)
    Surgi-Stim postsurgical
      therapy system
    UlcerJet system
    VAPR arthroscopic system

system (*continued*)
    X-PRESS vascular closure
      system
    Zephir anterior cervical
      plate (ACP) system

T

table
> AlphaStar operating room t.
> Andrews spinal surgery t.
> Stryker fracture t.

Tactilaze angioplasty laser catheter

Takahashi
> T. cutting forceps
> T. ethmoidal forceps

Taka microneurosurgical sponge

Takumi PTCA catheter

Talent
> T. endoluminal stent-graft system
> T. LPS endoluminal stent-graft system

T-Anastaflo shunt

TandemHeart ventricular assist device

Tanne corneal punch

Tanner mesher

Tanner-Vandeput mesh dermatome

tantalum
> t. mesh
> t. plate
> t. ring
> t. wire

tape
> Cath-Secure hypoallergenic
> CollaTape t.
> Dacron
> Deknatel would closure t.
> Elastikon elastic t.
> Hypafix t.
> Hy-T.
> Microfoam surgical t.
> Shur-Strip t.
> Transpore surgical t.

Taut
> T. catheter
> T. cystic duct c.

Techstar percutaneous closure device

Tegaderm transparent dressing

Tegagel hydrogel dressing

Tegagen alginate wound dressing

Tegapore contact-layer wound dressing

Tegasorb dressing

tenaculum
> Abel-Aesculap-Pratt t.
> Braun uterine t.
> Cottle single-prong t.
> lion jaw t.

Tenckhoff peritoneal dialysis catheter

Tennis Racquet catheter

Terry-Mayo needle

Terumo guide wire

The Closer arterial closure device

Therastream microcatheter

ThermaChoice Uterine Balloon Therapy

Therma Jaw hot urologic forceps

ThermoFX mesh

TherOx infusion guide wire

THI needle

THINSite
> T. dressing
> T. with BioFilm hydrogel topical wound dressing

Thomas
    T. needle
    T. shunt
    T. splint

Thoralon biomaterial

Thora-Port

Thoratec Heartmate left
    ventricular assist system
    (LVAS)

Thrombo-gard

Ti-Cron suture

Tielle absorptive dressing

TiMesh titanium mesh bone-
    plate and screw system

Tischler cervical biopsy punch
    forceps

Tisseel fibrin sealant

TissueLink monopolar floating
    ball

tissue morcellator

Titan
    T. ArthroWand
    T. Mega PTCA dilatation
        catheter
    T. Mega XL PTCA dilatation
        catheter

TomCat PTCA guide wire

Tourguide guiding catheter

Tracer over-the-wire
    intravascular mapping
    catheter

traction
    Bryant's t.
    Buck's t.
    Cotrel t.
    Crutchfield skeletal t.
    halo t.
    halter t.
    Russell's t.

Transeal transparent adhesive
    film dressing

TransiGel hydrogel-impregnated
    gauze

TrapEase

TraumaSeal topical wound
    closure device

transluminal extraction catheter

Transorbent multilayer dressing

Treace Tytan ventilation tube

Trelex mesh

trephine
    Barron disposable t.
    Barron radial vacuum t.

Trident
    T. resection ablator
    T. Omega blade

TriFix spinal instrumentation
    system

Trilogy
    T. acetabular cup
    T. DC+pacemaker
    T. SR+single-chamber
        pacemaker

Trippi-Wells tongs

Triumph VR pacemaker

Trocan disposable CO_2 trocar

trocar
    Abelson cricothyrotomy t.
    Bluntport disposable t.
    pyramidal tip t.

Tru-Close wound drainage
    system

Tru-Cut needle

True/Fit femoral intramedullary
    rod system

True/Flex intramedullary rod
    system

True/Lok external fixator system

T-Span tissue expander

tube
    Abbott t.
    Abbott-Rawson
        gastrointestinal double-
        lumen t.
    AccuMark calibrated infant
        feeding t.
    Activent ear t.
    Adson aspirating t.
    Adson brain suction t.
    Adson neurosurgical
        suction t.
    Air-Lon laryngectomy t.
    Air-Lon tracheal t.
    Aire-Cuf endotracheal t.
    Aire-Cuf tracheostomy t.
    Alesen t.
    American circle
        nephrostomy t.
    American Heyer-Schulte T-t.
    Amersham J t.
    Andersen mercury-
        weighted t.
    Anderson flexible suction t.
    Andrews-Pynchon suction t.
    angled pleural t.
    anode t.
    Anthony aspirating t.
    Anthony mastoid suction t.
    Anthony suction t.
    antifog t.
    aortic sump t.
    Argyle chest t.
    Argyle endotracheal t.
    Argyle Sentinel Seal chest t.
    Argyle-Dennis t.
    Armstrong beveled
        grommet drain t.
    Armstrong beveled
        grommet myringotomy t.
    Armstrong V-Vent t.
    Armstrong ventilation t.
    Arrow t.
    Asepto suction t.
    aspirating t.

tube (*continued*)
    Aspisafe nasogastric t.
    t. attachment device
    Atkins-Cannard
        tracheotomy t.
    auditory tube
    Ayre t.
    Baerveldt glaucoma
        implant t.
    Baerveldt shunt t.
    Baker jejunostomy t.
    Baker self-sumping t.
    Baldwin butterfly
        ventilation t.
    Bard gastrostomy feeding t.
    Bard PEG t.
    Bardic t.
    Barnes suction t.
    Baron ear t.
    Baron suction t.
    Baron-Frazier suction t.
    Baylor cardiovascular
        sump t.
    Baylor intracardiac sump t.
    Beall-Feldman-Cooley
        sump t.
    Beardsley empyema t.
    Bel-O-Pak suction t.
    Bellocq t.
    Bellucci suction t.
    Ben-Jet t.
    Benjamin t.
    Bettman empyema t.
    bicanalicular silicone t.
    Billroth t.
    Biolite ventilation t.
    Biosystems feeding t.
    Bivona Fome-Cuf t.
    Bivona Medical
        Technologies customized
        tracheostomy t.
    Bivona sleep apnea
        tracheostomy t.
    Bivona TTS tracheostomy t.
    bladder flap t.
    Blakemore esophageal t.
    Blakemore nasogastric t.
    Blakemore-Sengstaken t.

tube (*continued*)
  Blue Line cuffed
    endotracheal t.
  blunt suction t.
  bobbin myringotomy t.
  Bonney uterine t.
  Bouchut laryngeal t.
  Bourdon t.
  Bower PEG t.
  Bowman t.
  Brawley nasal suction t.
  bronchial t.
  Broncho-Cath double-
    lumen endotracheal t.
  bronchoscopy disposable
    suction t.
  Bruecke t.
  Bucy suction t.
  Bucy-Frazier suction t.
  Buie rectal suction t.
  Butler tonsillar suction t.
  Buyes air-vent suction t.
  calibrated grasping t.
  calix t.
  Caluso PEG gastrostomy t.
  Cantor intestinal t.
  capillary t.
  Carabelli endobronchial t.
  Carden bronchoscopy t.
  Carden laryngoscopy t.
  Carl Zeiss myringotomy t.
  Carlens double-lumen
    endotracheal t.
  Carman rectal t.
  Carrel t.
  Casselberry sphenoid t.
  Castelli-Paparella collar
    button t.
  cathode ray tube CRT
  Cattell forked-type T- t.
  Cattell gallbladder t.
  Celestin endoesophageal t.
  Celestin latex rubber t.
  t. changer
  Chaoul voltage x-ray t.
  Charnley drain t.
  Chauffin-Pratt t.
  Chaussier t.

tube (*continued*)
  chest t.
  Chevalier Jackson tracheal
    t.
  ClearCut II with smoke
    eater t.
  Clerf laryngectomy t.
  closed-suction t.
  coagulation suction t.
  coagulation-aspirator t.
  Coakley wash t.
  Cole endotracheal t.
  Cole orotracheal t.
  Cole pediatric t.
  Cole uncuffed endotracheal
    t.
  collar-button t.
  collecting t.
  Colton empyema t.
  Combitube endotracheal t.
  Comfit endotracheal t.
  Compat surgical feeding t.
  Cone suction t.
  Cone-Bucy suction t.
  conical centrifuge t.
  Connell breathing t.
  Connell ether vapor t.
  Contigen t.
  continuous suction t.
  Cook County Hospital
    tracheal suction t.
  Cooley aortic sump t.
  Cooley cardiovascular
    suction t.
  Cooley graft suction t.
  Cooley intracardiac suction
    t.
  Cooley sump suction t.
  Cooley vascular suction t.
  Cooley-Anthony suction t.
  Coolidge tube
  Cope loop nephrostomy t.
  corneal t.
  Corpak weighted-tip, self-
    lubricating t.
  Costen suction t.
  Cottle suction t.
  Coupland nasal suction t.

tube (*continued*)
Crawford t.
cricothyrotomy trocar t.
Crookes-Hittorf tube
cuffed endotracheal t.
cuffed tracheostomy t.
CUI myringotomy t.
Dakin t.
Dandy suction t.
David
  pharyngolaryngectomy t.
Davol t.
Dawson-Yuhl suction t.
Dean wash t.
Deane t.
Deaver t.
DeBakey suction t.
DeBakey-Adson suction t.
Debove t.
Denker t.
Dennis t.
DePaul t.
Devers gall bladder t.
DeVilbiss suction t.
Devine-Millard-Frazier
  fiberoptic suction t.
diagnostic t.
DIC tracheostomy t.
digestive tube
digit t.
disposable Yankauer
  aspirating t.
disposable Yankauer
  suction t.
Dobbhoff gastrectomy
  feeding t.
Dobbhoff gastric
  decompression t.
Dobbhoff nasogastric
  feeding t.
Dobbhoff PEG t.
Doesel-Huzly
  bronchoscopic t.
Donaldson drain t.
Donaldson eustachian t.
Donaldson myringotomy t.
Donaldson ventilation t.
double setup endotracheal t.

tube (*continued*)
double-cannula
  tracheostomy t.
double-focus t.
double-lumen
  endobronchial t.
double-lumen suction
  irrigation t.
doughnut tip suction t.
Dr. Bruecke aspirating t.
Dr. Twiss duodenal t.
drain-to-wall suction t.
t. dressing
dual-lumen sump
  nasogastric t.
Duke t.
Dundas-Grant t.
Duralite t.
Durham tracheostomy t.
Dynamic digit extensor t.
E. Benson Hood
  Laboratories esophageal t.
E. Benson Hood
  Laboratories salivary
  bypass t.
Eastman suction t.
EDTA-Vacutainer t.
Einhorn t.
electron multiplier t.
Endo-Tube nasal jejunal
  feeding t.
endobrachial double-lumen
  t.
endobronchial tube
endoesophageal t.
Endosoft reinforced cuffed
  t.
endotracheal tube
Endotrol endotracheal t.
enteroclysis t.
enterolysis t.
EntriStar feeding t.
EntriStar percutaneous
  endoscopic gastrostomy
  (PEG) t.
Eppendorf t.
ESKA-Buess esophageal t.
Esmarch t.

tube (*continued*)
    ET t.
    Ethox rectal t.
    eustachian tube
    Ewald t.
    extension t.
    Fay suction t.
    feeding tube
    fenestrated tracheostomy t.
    Ferguson-Frazier suction t.
    Feuerstein drainage t.
    Feuerstein split ventilation t.
    fiberoptic suction t.
    field emission tube
    fil D'Arion silicone t.
    Finsterer myringotomy split
        t.
    Finsterer suction t.
    Fitzpatrick suction t.
    flanged Teflon t.
    Flexiflo enteral feeding t.
    Flexiflo Inverta-PEG t.
    Flexiflo Sacks-Vine t.
    Flexiflo Stomate low-profile
        gastrostomy t.
    Flexiflo suction feeding t.
    Flexiflo tap-fill enteral t.
    Flexiflo Taptainer t.
    Flexiflo tungsten-weighted
        feeding t.
    Flexiflo Versa-PEG t.
    flow regulated suction t.
    fluffy-cuffed t.
    t. foam
    Fome-Cuf endotracheal t.
    Fome-Cuf pediatric
        tracheostomy t.
    Franco triflange ventilation t.
    Frazier aspirating t.
    Frazier brain suction t.
    Frazier Britetrac nasal
        suction t.
    Frazier fiberoptic suction t.
    Frazier modified suction t.
    Frazier nasal suction t.
    Frazier suction t.
    Frazier-Ferguson aspirating
        t.

tube (*continued*)
    Frazier-Ferguson ear
        suction t.
    Frazier-Paparella mastoid
        suction t.
    Frederick-Miller t.
    frontal sinus wash t.
    Fuller bivalve trach t.
    Gabriel Tucker t.
    gastric t.
    Gastro-Port II feeding t.
    gastrojejunostomy t.
    gastrostomy feeding t.
    Gavriliu gastric t.
    Geiger-Müller tube
    Gillquist suction t.
    Gillquist-Stille arthroplasty
        suction t.
    Glover suction t.
    glutaraldehyde-tanned
        bovine collagen t.
    Gomco suction t.
    Goode T-t.
    Goode T-tube ventilating t.
    Goode Trim t.
    Goodhill-Pynchon tonsillar
        suction t.
    Gott t.
    Gowen decompression t.
    Grafco Martin laryngectomy
        t.
    t. graft
    graft suction t.
    Great Ormond Street
        pediatric tracheostomy t.
    Greiling gastroduodenal t.
    grommet drain t.
    grommet myringotomy t.
    grommet ventilating t.
    Guibor Silastic t.
    Guilford-Wright suction t.
    Guisez t.
    Gwathmey suction t.
    Haering t.
    Hagan surface suction t.
    Hakim t.
    Haldane tube
    Haldane-Priestly t.

tube (*continued*)

Har-el pharyngeal t.
Hardy suction t.
Heimlich t.
Heimlich-Gavrilu gastric t.
Helsper tracheostomy vent t.
Hemagard collection t.
Hemovac suction t.
heparin-bonded Bott-type t.
Herring t.
Hi-Lo Jet tracheal t.
Holinger open-end aspirating t.
Holter t.
Hossli suction t.
hot cathode x-ray t.
Hotchkiss ear suction t.
Hough-Cadogan suction t.
House endolymphatic shunt t.
House suction t.
House-Baron suction t.
House-Radpour suction t.
House-Stevenson suction t.
House-Urban t.
Houser cul-de-sac irrigator t.
Hubbard airplane vent t.
Hugly aspirating t.
Humphrey coronary sinus-sucker suction t.
Hunsaker jet ventilation t.
Hymlek portable chest t.
Hyperflex tracheostomy t.
image Orthicon t.
Immergut suction t.
Immergut suction-coagulation t.
infusion t.
intracardiac suction t.
intracardiac sump t.
Isolator lysis-centrifugation t.
Israel suction t.
J-shaped t.
Jackson aspirating t.
Jackson cane-shaped tracheal t.

tube (*continued*)

Jackson cone-shaped tracheal t.
Jackson laryngectomy t.
Jackson open-end aspirating t.
Jackson silver tracheostomy t.
Jackson tracheal t.
Jackson velvet-eye aspirating t.
Jackson warning stop t.
Jackson-Pratt suction t.
Jackson-Rees endotracheal t.
Jacques gastric t.
Jako laryngeal suction t.
Jako laser aspirating t.
Jako suction t.
Jarit-Poole abdominal suction t.
Jarit-Yankauer suction t.
Javid bypass t.
jejunal feeding t.
Jesberg aspirating t.
Jiffy t.
Johnson coagulation suction t.
Johnson intestinal t.
Jones Pyrex t.
Jones tear duct t.
Jutte t.
K-Tube t.
Kangaroo silicone gastrostomy feeding t.
Kaslow gastrointestinal t.
Kay-Cross suction tip suction t.
Kehr gallbladder t.
Kelly t.
Keofeed feeding t.
KeyMed esophageal t.
Kidd U-t.
Killian t.
Kistner plastic tracheostomy t.
Klein ventilation t.
Knoche t.

tube (*continued*)
   Kos ear suction t.
   Kozlowski t.
   Kuhn endotracheal t.
   Kurze suction t.
   L.T. Jones tear duct t.
   Lacor t.
   Lahey Y-tube t.
   Lanz low-pressure cuff
      endotracheal t.
   Lanz tracheostomy t.
   Lar-A-Jext laryngectomy t.
   LaRocca nasolacrimal t.
   Laryngoflex reinforced
      endotracheal t.
   Laser-Shield XII wrapped
      endotracheal t.
   Laser-Trach endotracheal t.
   Lasertubus tracheal t.
   Leiter t.
   Lell tracheal t.
   Lenard ray t.
   Lennarson t.
   Lepley-Ernst tracheal t.
   Lester Jones t.
   Levin duodenal t.
   Levin-Davol t.
   Lewis laryngectomy t.
   Lezius suction t.
   life-saving t.
   Lindeman-Silverstein Arrow
      t.
   Lindeman-Silverstein
      ventilation t.
   Lindholm tracheal t.
   Linton esophageal t.
   Linton-Nachlas t.
   Lo-Por tracheal t.
   Lonnecken t.
   Lord-Blakemore t.
   Lore suction t.
   Lore-Lawrence
      tracheotomy t.
   Luer speaking t.
   Luer tracheal t.
   Lukens collecting t.
   Lyon t.
   McGowan-Keeley t.

tube (*continued*)
   Mackler intraluminal t.
   Mackray short-cuffed
      endobronchial t.
   McMurtry-Schlesinger shunt
      t.
   Magill Safety Clear
      endotracheal t.
   Maingot gallbladder t.
   Malecot nephrostomy t.
   Malis-Frazier suction t.
   malleable multipore
      suction t.
   Mallinckrodt endotracheal t.
   Mallinckrodt Laser-Flex t.
   Martin laryngectomy t.
   Martin tracheostomy t.
   Mason suction t.
   Massie sliding nail t.
   mastoid suction t.
   Mead Johnson t.
   mediastinal t.
   Medina t.
   Medoc-Celestin t.
   mesh myringotomy t.
   Methodist vascular suction
      t.
   Mett t.
   MIC bolus gastrostomy t.
   MIC gastroenteric t.
   MIC jejunal t.
   MIC jejunostomy t.
   MIC-Key gastrostomy t.
   microbore Tygon t.
   Microfuge t.
   Microgel surface-enhanced
      ventilation t.
   microlaryngeal
      endotracheal t.
   Micron bobbin ventilation t.
   Mill-Rose t.
   Miller endotracheal t.
   Miller-Abbott double-lumen
      intestinal t.
   Millin suction t.
   Milroy-Piper suction t.
   Minnesota t.
   Mixter t.

tube (*continued*)

modified suction t.
Molteno shunt t.
molybdenum rotating-anode x-ray t.
molybdenum target tube
Momberg t.
Montando t.
Montefiore tracheal t.
Montgomery esophageal t.
Montgomery salivary bypass t.
Montgomery T-t.
Montgomery tracheal t.
Moore t.
Morch swivel tracheostomy t.
Moretz Tiny Tytan ventilation t.
Moretz Tytan ventilation t.
Morse suction t.
Morse-Andrews suction t.
Morse-Ferguson suction t.
Mosher intubation t.
Mosher life-saving tracheal suction t.
Moss balloon triple-lumen gastrostomy t.
Moss feeding t.
Moss gastric decompression t.
Moss gastrostomy t.
Moss Mark IV t.
Moss nasal t.
Moss Suction Buster t.
Moss suction buster t.
Moulton lacrimal duct t.
Mousseau-Barbin esophageal t.
Mueller suction t.
Mueller-Frazier suction t.
Mueller-Poole suction t.
Mueller-Pynchon suction t.
Mueller-Yankauer suction t.
Muldoon t.
muscular t.
Myerson wash t.
myringotomy drain t.

tube (*continued*)

Nachlas gastrointestinal t.
Nachlas-Linton t.
nasal suction t.
nasobiliary t.
nasocystic drainage t.
nasoendotracheal t.
nasoenteric feeding t.
nasogastric feeding t.
nasoileal t.
nasojejunal t.
nasotracheal tube
NCC Hi-Lo Jet endotracheal t.
nephrostomy tube
Neuber bone t.
New Luer-type speaking t.
New speaking t.
New York glass suction t.
Newvicon camera t.
Newvicon vacuum chamber pickup t.
NG feeding t.
Nilsson suction t.
Nilsson-Stille abortion suction t.
Nishizaki-Wakabayashi suction t.
Norton endotracheal t.
Nunez ventricular ventilation t.
Nuport PEG t.
Nyhus-Nelson gastric decompression t.
Nyhus-Nelson jejunal feeding t.
Nystroem abdominal suction t.
O'Beirne sphincter t.
obstructed shunt t.
Ochsner gallbladder t.
O'Dwyer tube
O'Hanlon-Poole suction t.
Olshevsky t.
Olympus One-Step Button gastrostomy t.
Ommaya ventricular t.
opaque myringotomy t.

tube (*continued*)
    open-end aspirating t.
    oral endotracheal t.
    oral esophageal t.
    oroendotracheal t.
    orogastric Ewald t.
    orotracheal tube
    Ossoff-Karlan laser suction
       t.
    overcouch t.
    Oxford nonkinking cuffed t.
    Panda gastrostomy t.
    Panda nasoenteric feeding
       t.
    Panje t.
    Paparella myringotomy t.
    Paparella type II ventilation
       t.
    Paparella-Frazier suction t.
    Parker t.
    Paul intestinal drainage t.
    Paul-Mixter t.
    pear-shaped extension t.
    Pedia-Trake t.
    Pee Wee low-profile
       gastrostomy t.
    PEG tube, percutaneous
       endoscopic gastrostomy t.
    Penrose t.
    Per-Lee equalizing t.
    Per-Lee myringotomy t.
    Per-Lee ventilation t.
    percutaneous nephrostomy
       t.
    Perspex t.
    Pertrach percutaneous
       tracheostomy t.
    pharyngotympanic t.
    photoelectric multiplier t.
    photomultiplier tube
    pickup t.
    Pierce antrum wash t.
    pigtail nephrostomy t.
    Pilling duralite t.
    Pitot tube
    Pitt talking tracheostomy t.
    plastic-cuffed tracheostomy
       t.

tube (*continued*)
    Pleur-evac suction t.
    pleural t.
    Plumicon camera t.
    Polisar-Lyons adapted
       tracheal t.
    Polisar-Lyons tracheal t.
    polyethylene t.
    polyvinyl chloride
       endotracheal t.
    Ponsky PEG t.
    Ponsky-Gauderer PEG t.
    Poole abdominal suction t.
    Poppen suction t.
    Portex Blue Line
       tracheostomy t.
    Portex Per-Fit tracheostomy
       t.
    Portex preformed blue line
       tracheal t.
    Porto-Vac suction t.
    postpyloric feeding t.
    preformed polyvinyl
       chloride endotracheal t.
    pressure equalization t.
    pressure equalizing t.
    Pribram suction t.
    primordial catheter t.
    Proctor suction t.
    Pudenz t.
    Puestow-Olander
       gastrointestinal t.
    Pynchon suction t.
    Questek laser t.
    Quincke t.
    Quinton t.
    Radius enteral feeding t.
    Radpour-House suction t.
    RAE endotracheal t.
    RAE-Flex tracheal t.
    Rand-House suction t.
    Rand-Radpour suction t.
    rectal t.
    rectifier tube
    red rubber endotracheal t.
    Redivac suction t.
    Rehfuss duodenal t.
    Rehfuss stomach tube

tube (*continued*)

Reinecke-Carroll lacrimal t.
reinforced tracheostomy t.
Replogle t.
Reuter bobbin ventilation t.
Rhoton-Merz suction t.
Rica mastoid suction t.
right-angle chest t.
Ring-McLean sump t.
Ritter suprapubic suction t.
Robertshaw tube
Robinson equalizing t.
Rochester suction t.
Rochester tracheal t.
Roller pump suction t.
Rosen suction t.
rotating anode tube
Rusch laryngectomy t.
Rusch red rubber rectal t.
Ruschelit polyvinyl chloride
    endotracheal t.
Russell suction t.
Ryle duodenal t.
Sachs suction t.
Sacks-Vine PEG t.
Safety Clear Plus
    endotracheal t.
Salem sump action
    nasogastric t.
salivary bypass t.
Samco t.
Samson-Davis infant
    suction t.
Sandoz balloon
    replacement t.
Sandoz Caluso PEG
    gastrostomy t.
Sandoz feeding/suction t.
Sandoz nasogastric feeding
    t.
Sandoz suction t.
Sandoz suction/feeding t.
Sapporo shunt t.
Sarns intracardiac suction t.
Saticon vacuum chamber
    pickup t.
scavenging t.
Schall laryngectomy t.

tube (*continued*)

Schmiedt t.
Schuknecht suction t.
Schuler aspiration/irrigation
    t.
Scott nasal suction t.
Scott-Harden t.
Securat suction t.
Sengstaken nasogastric t.
Sengstaken-Blakemore
    esophagogastric
    tamponade t.
Sensiv endotracheal t.
separator t.
Seroma-Cath drainage t.
Seroma-Cath feeding t.
Shah myringotomy t.
Shah permanent
    ventilation t.
Shea-type parasol
    myringotomy t.
Sheehy collar-button
    ventilating t.
Sheehy Tytan
    ventilation t.
Shepard drain t.
Shepard grommet
    ventilation t.
Sherman suction t.
Shiley cuffless fenestrated t.
Shiley cuffless
    tracheostomy t.
Shiley disposable cannula
    low pressure cuffed
    tracheostomy t.
Shiley extra-length single
    cannula tracheostomy t.
Shiley fenestrated low
    pressure cuffed
    tracheostomy t.
Shiley French sump t.
Shiley laryngectomy t.
Shiley low-pressure cuffed
    tracheostomy t.
Shiley neonatal
    tracheostomy t.
Shiley pediatric
    tracheostomy t.

tube (*continued*)

  Shiley single cannula cuffed
      tracheostomy t.
  Silastic eustachian t.
  Silastic intestinal t.
  Silastic sucker suction t.
  Silastic tracheostomy t.
  silicone t.
  silicone-lubricated
      endotracheal t.
  Silverstein permanent
      aeration t.
  Singer-Blom t.
  siphon suction t.
  SMIC mastoid suction t.
  Smith t.
  smoke evacuator suction t.
  smoke removal t.
  Smokeeter t.
  Snyder Hemovac suction t.
  Snyder Surgivac suction t.
  Snyder Urevac suction t.
  Softech endotracheal t.
  SoftForm t.
  Soileau Tytan ventilation t.
  solid-phase extraction t.
  Southey capillary drainage
      t.
  Souttar t.
  speaking tube
  Spetzler MicroVac suction t.
  spiral-wound endotracheal
      t.
  SS bobbin drain t.
  SS bobbin myringotomy t.
  Stamm gastrostomy t.
  Stedman continuous
      suction t.
  stomach tube
  Stomate decompression t.
  Stomate extension t.
  Storz suction t.
  straight chest t.
  Stroud-Baron ear suction t.
  suction t.
  suction-coagulation t.
  Suh ventilation t.
  sump t.

tube (*continued*)

  Super PEG t.
  Sustagen nasogastric t.
  Swan-Ganz t.
  Swenson cholangiography
      t.
  T self-retaining drainage t.
  T-grommet ventilation t.
  T-tube round suction t.
  T-type myringotomy t.
  tear duct t.
  Thal-Quick chest t.
  Thora-Klex chest t.
  thoracostomy tube
  tight-to-shaft Aire-Cuf
      tracheostomy t.
  Tiny Tytan ventilation t.
  Tiny-Tef ventilation t.
  tonsillar suction t.
  Touma T-type grommet
      ventilation t.
  Tovell tube
  Toynbee diagnostic t.
  tracheal tube
  TracheoSoft XLT
      tracheostomy t.
  tracheostomy tube
  TRACOEflex tracheostomy
      t.
  Trake-Fit endotracheal t.
  translucent drain t.
  translucent myringotomy t.
  transpyloric feeding t.
  Trombotect t.
  TTS Aire-Cuf endotracheal
      t.
  TTS Aire-Cuf tracheostomy
      t.
  Tucker aspirating t.
  Tucker flexible-tip t.
  Tucker tracheal t.
  Turkel t.
  Turner-Warwick fiberoptic
      suction t.
  Turner-Warwick
      illuminating suction t.
  twist-in drain t.
  twist-in myringotomy t.

tube (*continued*)
    tympanostomy tube
    Tytan grommet ventilation t.
    Tytan ventilation t.
    U-tube t.
    underwater-seal suction t.
    Univent endotracheal t.
    urinary drainage t.
    uterine tube
    Vacutainer vacuum t.
    Valentine irrigation t.
    Van Alyea antral wash t.
    vascular suction t.
    velvet-eye aspirating t.
    Venturi bobbin myringotomy t.
    Venturi collar-button myringotomy t.
    Venturi grommet myringotomy t.
    Venturi pediatric myringotomy t.
    Vernon antral wash t.
    Versatome laser fiber t.
    Vidicon camera t.
    Vidicon vacuum chamber pickup t.
    Vinyon-N cloth t.
    Vivonex gastrostomy t.
    Voltolini ear t.
    Von Eichen antral wash t.
    Vortex tracheotomy t.
    Wangensteen duodenal t.
    Wannagat suction t.
    water-seal chest t.
    Webster infusion t.
    Weck coagulating suction t.
    Weck suction t.
    Welch Allyn suction t.
    Wendl t.
    Wepsic suction t.
    Williams esophageal t.
    Wilson-Cook nasobiliary t.
    Wilson-Cook NJFT-series feeding t.

tube (*continued*)
    Winsburg-White bladder t.
    Wolf suction t.
    Woodbridge t.
    woven Dacron t.
    Wullstein microsuction t.
    Xomed endotracheal t.
    Xomed straight-shank t.
    Xomed Treace ventilation t.
    Xomed Tytan ventilation t.
    x-ray tube
    Yankauer aspirating t.
    Yankauer suction t.
    Yasargil microsuction t.
    Yasargil suction t.
    Yeder suction t.
    Z-wave t.
    Zollner suction t.
    Zyler t.

tubing forceps

tumescent absorbent bandage dressing

Tuohy needle

Tupper retractor

TurboVac ArthroWand

Tutofix pin

Twisk
    T. forceps
    T. needle holder
    T. scissors

Tycron suture

Tygon tubing

Tylok high-tension cerclage cabling system

Typhoon microdebrider blade

Tytan ventilation tube

T-Y stent

U

UlcerJet system

Ulson fixation system

Ultimax distal femoral intramedullary rod system

UltraCision ultrasonic knife

Ultra-Drive bone cement removal system

UltraEdge keratome blade

Ultra 8 balloon catheter

Ultrafera wound dressing

Ultraflex stent

UltraKlenz wound cleanser

UltraLite flow-directed microcatheter

Ultratome

Uniflex intramedullary femoral nail system

Unigraft bone graft material

Unilab Surgibone

UNILINK system

Unimar J-Needle

UniShaper single-use keratome

Universal fixation screw

Unna-Flex compression dressing

Unna paste

unreamed femoral nail

Upper Hands retractor

Ureflex ureteral catheter

UroCoil self-expanding stent

Uroloop

UroLume urethral stent

UroMax II catheter

UroQuest On-Command catheter

Utrata capsulorrhexis forceps

V

Valle hysteroscope

ValleyLab
V. laparoscope
V. electrosurgical
instruments

valve
Abrams-Lucas flap heart v.
ATS Open Pivot Bileaflet
Heart v.
Biocor v.
Capetown aortic prosthetic
v.
CryoLife-O'Brien stentless
porcine heart v.
CryoValve-SG v.
Edwards Prima Plus v.
Freestyle v.
Ionescu tri-leaflet v.
Mosaic heart
Orbis-Sigma cerebrospinal
fluid v.
Quattro mitral v.
Ross pulmonary porcine v.
Top-Hat supra-annular
aortic v.
Xenomedica prosthetic v.
Xenotech prosthetic v.

Vanguard III endovascular aortic
graft

van Loonen operating
keratoscope

Vannas capsulotomy scissors

VaporTrode roller electrode

VAPR arthroscopic system

Varidyne drain

Varigrip spine fixation system

VariLift spinal cage

VariSoft steerable guide wire

Vas-Cath

VascuCoil peripheral vascular
stent

Vascufil suture

VascuGuard vascular patch

VascuLink vascular access graft

Vascutek Gelseal vascular graft

VasoSeal hemostatic device

Vaso View balloon dissection
system

Vasoview Uniport endoscopic
vein harvest system

Vector
V. intertrochanteric nail
V. large-lumen guiding
catheter

Vectra vascular access graft

Veingard transparent dressing

Velocity stent

Venaflow vascular graft

Venaport coronary sinus guiding
catheter

Vena Teck LGM filter

venoscope
Landry vein light v.

Ventak
V. AICD pacemaker
V. AV III DR automatic
implantable cardioverter-
defibrillator
V. Mini II automatic
implantable cardioverter-
defibrillator
V. Prizm dual chamber
implantable defibrillator

Ventex dressing

ventilation-exchange bougie

Ventra catheter

Ventritex Angstrom MD implantable cardioverter-defibrillator

Ventrix True Tech ICP catheter

Verbatim balloon catheter

Verbrugge bone clamp

Veridian umbilical clamp

Veripath peripheral guiding catheter

VerreScope microlaparoscope

Versabond cement

Versalok low back fixation system

VersaPoint hysteroscopic fibroid removal system

Versaport trocar

VersaTack stapling device

Versatrac lumbar retractor

Viasorb wound dressing

Vickers ring-tip forceps

Vicryl Rapide suture

VideoHydro laparoscope

Vigilon dressing

Vigor pacemaker

Visa II PTCA catheter

Visi-Black surgical needle

Visica cryoablation system

Visijet hydrokeratome

Visilex mesh

Vision PTCA catheter

Visiport optical trocar system

Visitec
V. circular knife
V. crescent knife
V. EdgeAhead phaco slit knife
V. stiletto knife

Vistaflex biliary stent

Vistec x-ray detectable sponge

VISX
V. excimer laser
V. Star S2 excimer laser system

Vitatron
V. catheter electrode
V. Diamond pacemaker
V. Jade II SSI pacemaker
V. Legacy II pacemaker
V. Ruby II DDD pacemaker
V. Topaz II SSIR pacemaker

Vitesse catheter

VITEK fibrin sealant

vitrector probe

VNUS
V. Closure catheter
V. Restore catheter

Volkmann spoon

Voorhees needle

Voyager aortic IntraClusion device

Vozzle Vacu-Irrigator

Vueport balloon-occlusion guiding catheter

Wallach ZoomScope

Wallstent Monorail carotid stent

Walsham forceps

Was-Cath thromboarterectomy catheter

Waterfield needle

Waterlase Millennium laser system

Watzke Silicone sleeve

WaveWire guide wire

Wedeen wire passer

Weitlaner retractor

Whitacre spinal needle

Wholey wire

Wiktor
 W. GX Hepamed coated coronary stent system
 W. Prime coronary stent system

Wilson-Cook wire-guided sphincterotome

Wiltse
 W. pedical screw system
 W. rod

wire
 ACS microglide w.
 Amplatz torque w.
 Ancrofil clasp w.
 w. appliance
 atrial pacing w.
 auger w.
 Australian orthodontic w.
 Australian Special Plus w.
 Babcock stainless steel suture w.
 Baron suction tube-cleaning w.
 bayonet-point w.

wire (*continued*)
 beaded cerclage w.
 Bentson exchange straight guide w.
 Bentson floppy-tip guide w.
 Bentson-type Glidewire guide w.
 w. bivalve vaginal speculum
 Birtcher Hyfrecator cautery w.
 bone fixation w.
 braided w.
 brass w.
 Brooker w.
 Bunnell pull-out w.
 central core w.
 cerclage w.
 cesium-137 w.
 Charnley trochanter w.
 circumdential w.
 Coffin transpalatal w.
 coiled spiral pusher w.
 Commander PTCA w.
 Compere fixation w.
 Conceptus Robust guide w.
 control w.
 Cope w.
 Cordis Stabilizer marker w.
 Cragg Convertible w.
 Cragg FX w.
 Cragg infusion w.
 crenulated tantalum w.
 w. crimper
 Crozat orthodontic w.
 curved J-exchange w.
 w. cutter
 Dall-Miles cerclage w.
 delivery w.
 Dentaflex w.
 diathermy w.
 double keyhole loop w.
 w. drill
 w. driver
 Drummond w.
 E wildcat orthodontic w.

wire (*continued*)
    ear snare w.
    eel w.
    endocardial w.
    Eve-Neivert tonsillar w.
    extra-stiff Amplatz w.
    w. fixation bolt
    FlowWire Doppler guide w.
    Force w.
    w. frame spectacles
    Geenan Endotorque w.
    Gigli spiral saw w.
    Gilmer w.
    Glidewire Gold surgical
      guide w.
    Guidant guide w.
    w. guide
    Hahnenkratt orthodontic w.
    Hancock temporary cardiac
      pacing w.
    Hi-Per Flex exchange w.
    high-torque w.
    House piston w.
    HPC guide w.
    hydrophilic-coated guide w.
    intermaxillary w.
    interosseous w.
    intracoronary Doppler flow
      w.
    intravascular Doppler-
      tipped guide w.
    Isola w.
    Isotac pilot w.
    Ivy w.
    J exchange w.
    J-w.
    Jagwire w.
    Jarabak arch w.
    Johnson canaliculus w.
    K w.
    K-w.
    Katzen infusion w.
    Killip w.
    Kirschner boring w.
    Kirschner w. K wire, K-w.
    w. lid speculum
    ligature tie w.
    lingual w.

wire (*continued*)
    Linx extension w.
    w. loop
    w. loop stapes dilator
    Lunderquist coat hanger w.
    Luque cerclage w.
    Luque sublaminar w.
    magnet w.
    Markley orthodontic w.
    w. mandrin
    Medi-Tech w.
    w. mesh eye implant
    monofilament snare w.
    Monorail guide w.
    Mullan w.
    Mustang steerable guide w.
    nasal snare w.
    needle-knife w.
    Neivert-Eves tonsillar w.
    nitinol shape-memory alloy
      w.
    olive w.
    outrigger w.
    over-tying w.
    pacing w.
    w. passer
    w. probe
    Pathfinder w.
    PD orthodontic w.
    piston w.
    platinum w.
    Prima laser guide w.
    w. prosthesis-crimping
      forceps
    prosthesis smooth w.
    protector plus w.
    Puestow guide w.
    pusher w.
    Quadcat w.
    QuickSilver hydrophilic-
      coated guide w.
    RadiMedical fiberoptic
      pressure-monitoring w.
    rectal cautery w.
    rectangular w.
    Remaloy w.
    Remanium w.
    Respond w.

wire (*continued*)
    Roadrunner w.
    Rotablator w.
    Rotafloppy w.
    round chuck-end Kirschner
        w.
    Sadowsky hook w.
    Sage w.
    w. saw
    Scimed-Choice floppy w.
    w. scissors
    Seldinger retrograde w.
    w. side blade
    Silk guide w.
    Simcoe anterior chamber
        retaining w.
    Sippy esophageal dilator
        pusher w.
    smooth transfixion w.
    snare w.
    w. snare
    space-age w.
    spinous process w.
    w. splint
    square w.
    stainless steel w.
    w. stapes prosthesis
    Sterling-Spring orthodontic
        w.
    Stertzer-Myler extension w.
    stiffening w.
    Storz twisted snare w.
    w. stylet
    w. stylet catheter
    sublaminar w.
    suture w.
    tantalum w.
    TherOx infusion guide w.
    Thiersch w.
    w. threader
    w. tightener

wire (*continued*)
    titanium w.
    tonsillar snare w.
    torque attenuating diameter
        w.
    Tracer ST w.
    Trailblazer w.
    trocar-point Kirschner w.
    trochanteric w.
    Truarch w.
    ultrastiff w.
    veneer retention w.
    Wholey w.
    Wildcat w.
    w. twister
    w. Zytor suture
    Wironit clasp w.
    Wirotom clasp w.
    Wizdom guide w.
    Zimaloy beaded suture w.

wishbone retractor

Wissinger rod

Wizard microdebrider

Wizdom guide wire

Wolvek sternal approximation
    fixation device

Workhorse PTCA balloon
    catheter

Woun'Dres hydrogel dressing

Wound-Span Bridge II dressing

Wrightlock posterior fixation
    system

Wright needle

Würzburg plating system

Wylie carotid artery clamp

X

Xact ACL graft-fixation system

XenoDerm graft

Xeroform gauze

Xia spinal system

Xomed
- X. Kartush insulated retractor
- X. Kartush typanic membrane patcher
- X. Tytan ventilation tube

Xpeedior catheter

X-PRESS vascular closure system

XPS Straightshot micro tissue resector

X-Sizer catheter system

XT coronary stent

XTRAC laser system

X-Trode stent

XXL balloon dilatation catheter

Y

Yankauer curette

Yasargil
    Y. bayonet scissors
    Y. permanent aneurysm clip

Yeoman uterine biopsy
    forceps

Yoon fallopian tube ligation
    ring

Z

Z-Clamp hysterectomy forceps

Zebra exchange guide wire

Zeiss
    Z. Endolive endoscoope
    Z. Visulas 690s laser

Zelsmyr Cytobrush

Zenith AAA endovascular graft system

Zephir anterior cervical plate (ACP) system

Zielke
    Z. curette
    Z. instrumentation

Zimmer Statak suture

Zinnanti Z-clamp

Ziramic femoral head

Zirconia orthopedic prosthetic head

Zone Specific II meniscal repair system

Z-Med catheter

ZMS intramedullary fixation system

Zoll defibrillator

Zone-Specific II meniscal repair system

Z-scissors hysterectomy scissors

Z-stent

ZTT acetabular cup

Zuma guiding catheter

ZUMI uterine manipulator

Zweymuller prosthesis